Clinical Significance and Potential of Selective COX-2 Inhibitors

The publishers are grateful to
Dr Michelle Browner,
Roche Bioscience, Palo Alto, California,
for the schematic diagram of the
human COX-2 dimer shown on the cover

Clinical Significance and Potential of Selective COX-2 Inhibitors

Edited by

JOHN R. VANE and REGINA M. BOTTING

The William Harvey Research Institute, Saint Bartholomew's Hospital Medical College, London, United Kingdom

The combined proceedings of the William Harvey Conferences held in Phuket, Thailand, on 18–19 September, 1997 and in Boston, USA, on 23–24 April, 1998, supported by an educational grant from

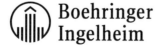

Boehringer
Ingelheim

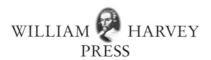

WILLIAM HARVEY
PRESS

Distributors

Gazelle Book Services Limited, Falcon House, Queen Square, Lancaster LA1 1RN.

A catalogue record for this book is available from the British Library.

ISBN 0 9534039 0 4

Copyright

Published in the United Kingdom by William Harvey Press, Saint Bartholomew's Hospital Medical College, Charterhouse Square, London EC1M 6BQ, UK.

Typeset by Cambridge Photosetting Services, Cambridge.

Printed and bound in Great Britain by MPG Books, Bodmin, Cornwall.

Contents

List of contributors

Phillip Bennett
Imperial College School of Medicine, Institute of Obstetrics and Gynaecology, Queen Charlottes and Chelsea Hospital, Goldhawk Road, London W6 OXG, UK.
Co-authors: Robert Sawdy, Donna Slater

Leslie J. Crofford
Department of Internal Medicine, Division of Rheumatology, University of Michigan, Room 5510E, MSRB I, 1150 West Medical Center Drive, Ann Arbor, MI 48109-0680, USA.

Raymond N. DuBois
Department of Medicine, Vanderbilt University Medical Center, 1161 21st Ave South, Nashville, TN 37232-2279, USA.
Co-authors: A. P. Goldman, C. S. Williams, L. W. Lamps, V. P. Williams, M. Pairet, J. D. Morrow

Helmut Fenner
Swiss Federal Institute of Technology, Zürich, Switzerland.

James F. Fries
Department of Medicine, Division of Immunology and Rheumatology, Stanford University School of Medicine, 1000 Welch Road, Suite 203, Palo Alto, CA 94304, USA.
Co-authors: Gurkirpal Singh, Dena R. Ramey

Christopher J. Hawkey
Department of Medicine, Division of Gastroenterology, University Hospital, Queen's Medical Centre, Nottingham NG7 2UH, UK.

David Henry
Discipline of Clinical Pharmacology, Faculty of Medicine and Health Sciences, Clinical Sciences Building, Mater Misericordiae Hospital, Waratah NSW 2298, Australia.
Co-authors: Patricia McGettigan, John Page

André Kahan
Division of Rheumatology, R. Descartes University, Hopital Cochin, 27 rue du Faubourg Saint-Jacques, 75679 Paris, Cedex 14, France.

John C. McGiff
Department of Pharmacology, New York Medical College, Basic Science Building, Rm 514, Valhalla, NY 10595, USA.
Co-authors: Nicholas R. Ferreri, Carlos P. Vio

M. Kerry O'Banion
Department of Neurobiology and Anatomy, University of Rochester Medical Center, 601 Elmwood Avenue, Box 603, Rochester, NY 14642, USA.

Michel Pairet
Department of Respiratory Research, Boehringer Ingelheim Research and Development, Birkendorfer Str. 65, 88397 Biberach a/d Riss, Germany.
Co-author: Joanne van Ryn

Carol C. Pilbeam
University of Connecticut Health Center, Farmington, CT 06030, USA.

Ari Ristimäki
Department of Obstetrics and Gynecology, Helsinki University Central Hospital and Department of Bacteriology and Immunology, The Haartman Institute, University of Helsinki, Haartmaninkatu 2, 00290 Helsinki, Finland.

Dirk O. Stichtenoth
Institute of Clinical Pharmacology, Hannover Medical School, Postfach 61 01 80, 30623 Hannover, Germany.
Co-author: Jürgen C. Frölich

Makoto M. Taketo
Laboratory of Biomedical Genetics, Graduate School of Pharmaceutical Sciences, University of Tokyo, 7-3-1 Hongo, Bunkyo-ku, Tokyo 113-0033, Japan.

John R. Vane
The William Harvey Research Institute, St Bartholomew's and the Royal London School of Medicine and Dentistry, Queen Mary and Westfield College, Charterhouse Square, London EC1M 6BQ, UK.
Co-author: Regina M. Botting

Brendan J. R. Whittle
The William Harvey Research Institute, St Bartholomew's and the Royal London School of Medicine and Dentistry, Queen Mary and Westfield College, Charterhouse Square, London EC1M 6BQ, UK.

M. Michael Wolfe
Section of Gastroenterology, Boston University School of Medicine and Boston Medical Center, 88 East Newton Street, Evans 201, Boston, MA 02118-2393, USA.
Co-author: Chi-Chuan Tseng

Preface

The therapy of rheumatism began thousands of years ago with the use of decoctions or extracts of herbs or plants such as willow bark or leaves, most of which turned out to contain salicylates. In the 1960s, the importance of a newly characterized group of lipid mediators called the prostaglandins in inflammation, fever and pain became evident. The discovery, by Vane in 1971, that all the chemically diverse members of the group of non-steroidal anti-inflammatory drugs (NSAIDs) acted by inhibiting the key enzyme in prostaglandin biosynthesis (which we now call cyclooxygenase or COX) provided a unifying explanation for their therapeutic actions and shared side effects. The clarification of the mode of action of the NSAIDs also gave the pharmaceutical industry a new tool for finding new drugs, using the COX enzyme in vitro as an initial screen. However, the side effects, especially on the stomach, were still a major problem and some companies began to look for new compounds which were anti-inflammatory, but were less damaging to the stomach. Meloxicam, now recognized as a selective COX-2 inhibitor, was discovered in this way.

The next important advance in our understanding of the NSAIDs came in 1991, when several laboratories showed that COX exists in two isomeric forms, COX-1 and COX-2. There is a constitutive isoform, COX-1, which has clear physiological functions. Its activation leads, for instance, to the production of prostacyclin which when released by the endothelium is antithrombogenic and when released by the gastric mucosa is cytoprotective. COX-1 in platelets produces thromboxane which promotes platelet aggregation and leads to thrombus formation. The second isoform is COX-2, which is inducible in a number of cells by pro-inflammatory stimuli. It is encoded by a different gene from COX-1. The amino acid sequence of its cDNA shows a 60% homology with the sequence of the non-inducible enzyme.

Since COX-2 is induced by inflammatory stimuli and by cytokines in migratory and other cells, it is attractive to suggest that the anti-inflammatory actions of NSAIDs are due to the inhibition of COX-2, whereas the unwanted side effects such as irritation of the stomach lining and toxic effects on the kidney are due to inhibition of the constitutive enzyme, COX-1. Clearly, to treat inflammation the NSAIDs will be used in doses that suppress COX-2. At such doses, the effects on COX-1 will vary according to the drug involved. Thus, drugs which have the highest potency on COX-2 and a better COX-2/COX-1 activity ratio will have potent anti-inflammatory activity with fewer side effects on the stomach and kidney. The COX-2/COX-1 ratios of a range of NSAIDs has been measured in several ways and the whole blood assay is now generally used. Results obtained with an improved whole blood assay show a strong correlation between the COX-2/COX-1 ratios and published figures of epidemiological data for gastric damage in humans, proving the concept that inhibition of COX-2 accounts for the anti-inflammatory actions of the NSAIDs, whereas inhibition of COX-1 causes the damage to the stomach mucosa.

The development of more selective inhibitors of COX-2 will clearly provide important advances in the therapy of inflammation. Conventional NSAIDs lead to gastrointestinal side effects, which include perforations, ulcerations and bleeds (PUBS) that lead to hospitalization of more than 100,000 patients a year in the USA alone. About 15% of these patients die in intensive care. The evidence is strong, both from animal tests and from the clinic that the selective COX-2 inhibitors will have greatly reduced side effects. Already, the extensive clinical trials comparing the gastric toxicity of meloxicam with that of diclofenac (MELISSA) and piroxicam (SELECT) have demonstrated the superior safety of meloxicam.

New uses will also be found for selective COX-2 inhibitors. For example, aspirin is effective in the prophylaxis of colon cancer and we now know that it is the induction of COX-2 that is associated with this condition. Selective COX-2 inhibitors, including meloxicam, prevent the growth of tumour cells in experimental carcinogenesis and some major drug companies have entered their compounds into clinical trials in colon cancer.

Also there is some less convincing evidence that Alzheimer's disease is associated with an upregulation of COX-2. It is thought that clinical trials with the lead COX-2 inhibitors have also been initiated.

COX-2 is induced during labour and initiates parturition, through producing prostaglandin $F_{2\alpha}$, which contracts the uterus. The selective COX-2 inhibitor, nimesulide, prevented pre-term labour in women who had already suffered several early abortions and meloxicam, with a longer half life, may well provide a better alternative.

This latest volume on the pharmacology of COX-2 discusses the current status of research into its pathophysiological functions in the synovium, bone, gastric mucosa and kidney. Results are presented of clinical trials with a selective COX-2 inhibitor (meloxicam) proving its advantages over standard NSAIDs. In addition, the role of COX-2 in colon cancer, parturition and Alzheimer's disease has been evaluated.

John R. Vane
Regina M. Botting

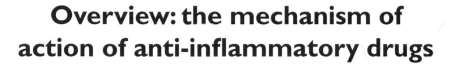

Overview: the mechanism of action of anti-inflammatory drugs

J. R. VANE AND R. M. BOTTING

Before 1971, many biochemical effects of the non-steroid anti-inflammatory drugs (NSAIDs) had been documented, and there were many hypotheses about their mode of action. It was observed, for example, that most of these drugs uncoupled oxidative phosphorylation[1] and that several salicylates inhibited dehydrogenase enzymes, especially those dependent upon pyridine nucleotides[2,3]. Some amino-transferases[4] and decarboxylases[5] were also inhibited and so were several key enzymes involved in protein and RNA biosynthesis[6]. However, the concentration of the drugs required for enzyme inhibition was in excess of the concentrations typically found in the plasma after therapy, and there was no convincing reason why inhibition of any of these enzymes should produce the triple anti-inflammatory, analgesic and antipyretic effects of aspirin.

THE PROSTAGLANDIN SYSTEM

It was against this background of knowledge that the investigation of the mode of action of NSAIDs was taken over by prostaglandin researchers. Piper and Vane employed the technique of continuous bioassay using the cascade bioassay system[7] developed by Vane in the mid-1960s for use with blood or an artificial salt solution.

Piper and Vane reported the anaphylactic release from isolated perfused lungs of the guinea pig of prostaglandins[8] and of another, very ephemeral, substance that was named 'rabbit aorta contracting substance' (RCS). In the lung perfusate RCS had a half life of about 2 minutes and it was identified in 1975 as thromboxane A_2 by Samuelsson's group[9]. The release of RCS from guinea pig isolated lungs during anaphylaxis was blocked by aspirin and similar drugs[10]. Vane postulated that the various stimuli which released prostaglandins were in fact 'turning on' the synthesis of these compounds and that aspirin might well be blocking their synthesis. Using the supernatant of a broken cell homogenate from guinea pig lung as a source of prostaglandin synthase, Vane found a dose-dependent inhibition of prostaglandin formation by aspirin, salicylate and indomethacin but not by morphine[11]. Two other reports from the same laboratory lent support to and extended his finding. Smith and Willis found that aspirin prevented the release of prostaglandins from aggregating human platelets[12] and Ferreira, Moncada and Vane demonstrated that aspirin-like drugs blocked prostaglandin release from the perfused, isolated spleen of the dog[13].

The discovery that all NSAIDs act by inhibiting the enzyme which we now call cyclooxygenase (COX), which leads to the generation of prostaglandins, provided a unifying explanation of their therapeutic actions and firmly established certain prostaglandins as important mediators of inflammatory disease (for reviews see references 14–16).

TWO ISOFORMS OF COX

Biochemistry

In 1976[17] COX, or prostaglandin endoperoxide synthase, with a molecular mass of 71 kDa was isolated, and it was cloned in 1988[18-20]. The enzyme exhibits both cyclooxygenase and hydroperoxidase activities. COX first cyclizes arachidonic acid to form prostaglandin G_2 and the peroxidase then reduces prostaglandin G_2 to prostaglandin H_2.

COX exists in at least two isoforms, COX-1 and COX-2. Garavito and his colleagues[21] have determined the three-dimensional structure of COX-1, which consists of three independent folding units: an epidermal growth factor-like domain, a membrane binding section and an enzymatic domain. The sites for peroxidase and cyclooxygenase activity are adjacent but spatially distinct. The enzyme integrates into only a single leaflet of the membrane lipid bilayer and thus the position of the cyclooxygenase channel allows arachidonic acid to gain access to the active site from the interior of the bilayer. Most NSAIDs compete with arachidonic acid for binding to the active site; uniquely, aspirin irreversibly inhibits COX-1 by acetylation of serine 530, thereby excluding access for the substrate[22].

The X-ray crystal structure of COX-2 closely resembles that of COX-1, but fortunately for the medicinal chemist, the binding sites for arachidonic acid on these enzymes are slightly different[23]. The active site of COX-2 is slightly larger and can accommodate bigger structures than those which are able to reach the active site of COX-1. A secondary internal pocket of COX-2 contributes significantly to the larger volume of the active site in this enzyme, although the central channel is also bigger by 17% (Figure 1).

Physiology

The constitutive isoform, COX-1, has clear physiological functions. Its activation leads, for instance, to the production of prostacyclin, which when released by the

Figure 1 (a) The structure of human COX-2. The COX-2 homodimer is represented by rendering the secondary structure elements; α-helices are depicted as cylinders, β-strands as thick arrows, connecting loops and turns by ribbons. The membrane binding domain is represented in white; the enzyme inhibitor occupying the cyclooxygenase active site is coloured green; the N-terminal EGF domain is shown in yellow and the haem moiety in the peroxidase active site in orange (reference 23). (b) Comparison of COX-2 and COX-1 NSAID binding sites. Representation of the accessible molecular surface at the binding site of flurbiprofen in the sheep COX-1 structure (reference 21), and of the inhibitor binding site in human COX-2 (reference 23). The pictures were generated using the program GRASP (Reproduced with permission of Michelle Browner).

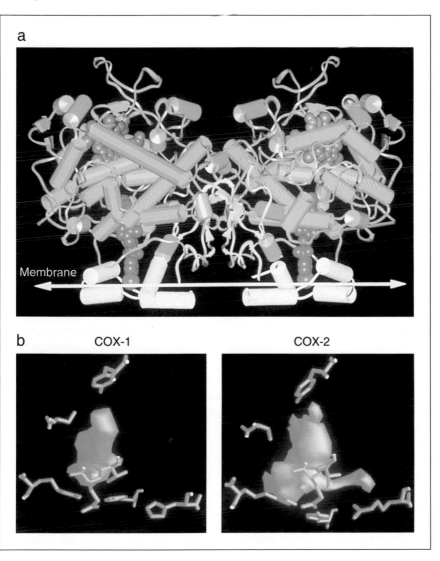

endothelium is antithrombogenic[24] and when released by the gastric mucosa is cytoprotective[25]. The inducible isoform, COX-2, was discovered some seven years ago and is induced in a number of cells by pro-inflammatory stimuli[26]. Its existence was first suspected when Needleman and his group reported that bacterial lipopolysaccharide (LPS) increased the synthesis of prostaglandins in human monocytes in vitro[27] and in mouse peritoneal macrophages in vivo[28]. This increase was inhibited by dexamethasone and associated with de novo synthesis of new COX protein. A year or so later, an inducible COX was identified as a distinct isoform of cyclooxygenase (COX-2) encoded by a different gene from COX-1[29–32]. Both enzymes have a molecular mass of 71 kDa and the amino acid sequence of the cDNA for COX-2 shows a 60% homology with the sequence of the non-inducible enzyme, with the size of the mRNA for the inducible enzyme approximating 4.5 kb and that of the constitutive enzyme being 2.8 kb. The inhibition by the glucocorticoids of the expression of COX-2 is an additional aspect of the anti-inflammatory action of the corticosteroids. The levels of COX-2, normally very low in cells, are tightly controlled by a number of factors, including cytokines and intracellular messengers, and by the availability of substrate.

Since COX-2 is induced by inflammatory stimuli and by cytokines in migratory and other cells it is attractive to suggest that the anti-inflammatory actions of NSAIDs are due to the inhibition of COX-2, whereas the unwanted side effects such as irritation of the stomach lining are due to inhibition of the constitutive enzyme, COX-1.

FUNCTIONS OF COX-1 AND COX-2

Gastrointestinal Tract

The so-called 'cytoprotective' action of prostaglandins in preventing gastric erosions and ulceration is mainly brought about by endogenously produced prostacyclin and prostaglandin E_2 (PGE_2), which reduce gastric acid secretion and exert a direct vasodilator action on the vessels of the gastric mucosa. In addition to these major actions, prostanoids stimulate the secretion of viscous mucus, gastric fluid and duodenal bicarbonate[33]. In most species, including humans, the bulk of the protective prostaglandins are synthesized by COX-1, although small quantities of COX-2 have been found in the normal rat stomach[34]. However, large quantities of COX-2 are expressed in experimentally induced and in human colon cancers[35,36].

It is at first puzzling why knockout mice in which the COX-1 gene has been deleted do not develop gastric ulcers spontaneously, but do show a decreased sensitivity to the damaging effects of indomethacin[37]. However, the normality of the mucosa in these mice could well be brought about by the continued release of nitric oxide and calcitonin gene-related peptide, both also known to contribute to the maintenance of a healthy mucosa[38]. The remaining ulcerogenic action of indomethacin may be caused by a local irritant effect on the gastric mucosal epithelium.

Kidney

Maintenance of kidney function both in animal models of disease states and patients with congestive heart failure, liver cirrhosis or renal insufficiency, is dependent on vasodilator prostaglandins. These patients are therefore at risk of renal ischaemia when prostaglandin synthesis is reduced by NSAIDs. Synthesis of PGE_2 and prostacyclin is mainly by COX-1 although low levels of mRNA for COX-2 have also been reported[39]. Upregulation of COX-2 expression has been observed in the macula densa following salt deprivation[39].

Mice that lack the gene for production of COX-1 appear to be perfectly healthy and do not show significant signs of kidney pathology. This is in accord with the finding that inhibition of COX-1 by NSAIDs does not alter renal function under normal physiological conditions. However, in COX-2 (−/−) null mice the kidneys failed to develop fully after birth with the result that the animals died before they were 8 weeks old[40].

Central Nervous System

COX-1 is found in neurones throughout the brain but it is most abundant in forebrain where prostaglandins may be involved in complex integrative functions such as control of the autonomic nervous system and in sensory processing[41,42]. COX-2 mRNA is induced in brain tissue and in cultured glial cells by pyrogenic substances such as LPS and interleukin (IL)-1[43,44]. However, low levels of COX-2 protein and COX-2 mRNA have been detected in neurones of the forebrain without previous stimulation by pro-inflammatory substances[41,42,45]. These 'basal' levels of COX-2 are particularly high in neonates and are probably induced by physiological nervous activity. Intense nerve stimulation, leading to seizures, induces COX-2 mRNA in discrete neurones of the hippocampus[46], whereas acute stress raises levels in the cerebral cortex[41]. COX-2 mRNA is also constitutively expressed in the spinal cord of normal rats and may be involved with processing of nociceptive stimuli[47]. Endogenous, fever-producing PGE_2 is thought to originate from COX-2 induced by LPS or IL-1 in endothelial cells lining the blood vessels of the hypothalamus[44]. The selective COX-2 inhibitor NS-398 is a potent antipyretic agent in rats[48].

Reproductive System

Expression of COX-1 is much greater than that of COX-2 in foetal hearts, kidneys, lungs and brains as well as in the decidual lining of the uterus[49,50]. Constitutive COX-1 in the amnion could also contribute prostaglandins for the maintenance of a healthy pregnancy[51]. In human amnion cells, chorionic gonadotrophin increases mRNA for COX-1[52], whereas glucocorticoids, epidermal growth factor, IL-1β and IL-4 all stimulate COX-2 expression[53,54]. Both COX-1 and COX-2 are expressed in the uterine epithelium at different times in early pregnancy and may be important for implantation of the ovum and for the angiogenesis necessary to establish the placenta[55].

Prostaglandins synthesized by COX-1 are apparently essential for the survival of foetuses during parturition, since the majority of offspring born to homozygous COX-1 knockout mice do not survive[37]. This high mortality of the pups may be due to premature closure of the ductus arteriosus. Female COX-2 knockout mice are mostly infertile, producing very few offspring due to a reduction in ovulation[56].

SELECTIVE INHIBITION OF COX-2

Sales of anti-inflammatory drugs are now estimated at 5.8 billion dollars a year with the USA accounting for 1.8 billion dollars (Scrip No. 2312, Feb 25 1998, p. 7). Yet they all have toxic effects on the stomach. Indeed, several epidemiological studies have characterized the degree of gastric damage caused by different compounds[57]. An estimated 34–46% of patients on NSAID therapy will have some form of gastrointestinal adverse events[58]. It is estimated that in the USA alone, some 80,000 patients on NSAIDs are hospitalized each year because of perforations, ulcers or bleeding (PUBs) in the stomach[59]. Some 10–20,000 of these patients die in intensive care. Of course, these hospitalizations only represent the extreme of gastric irritation, which ranges from mild dyspepsia all the way through to PUBs. Even ibuprofen, recognized as one of the mildest gastric irritants, causes problems in a significant proportion of patients. Clearly, there is dramatic need for anti-inflammatory drugs which do not affect the stomach.

The importance of the discovery of the inducible COX-2 is highlighted by the differences in pharmacology of the two enzymes[60]. Aspirin, indomethacin and ibuprofen are much less active against COX-2 than against COX-1[61]. Indeed, the strongest inhibitors of COX-1 such as aspirin, indomethacin and piroxicam are the NSAIDs which cause the most damage to the stomach[62]. The spectrum of activities of some ten standard NSAIDs against the two enzymes ranges from a high selectivity towards COX-1 (166-fold for aspirin) through to equiactivity on both[63].

The range of activities of NSAIDs against COX-1 compared with COX-2 explains the variations in the side effects of NSAIDs at their anti-inflammatory doses. Drugs which have a high potency against COX-2 and a low COX-2/COX-1 activity ratio will have potent anti-inflammatory activity with few side effects on the stomach and kidney. Garcia Rodriguez and Jick[64] have published a comparison of epidemiological data on the side effects of NSAIDs. Piroxicam and indomethacin in anti-inflammatory doses showed high gastrointestinal toxicity. These drugs have a much higher potency against COX-1 than against COX-2[65]. Thus, when epidemiological results are compared with COX-2/COX-1 ratios, there is a parallel relationship between gastrointestinal side effects and COX-2/COX-1 ratios.

Selective COX-2 Inhibitors in Current Therapeutic Use

Meloxicam, nimesulide and etodolac were identified in the 1980s as potent anti-inflammatory drugs with low ulcerogenic activity in the rat stomach. In some instances, this was also shown to parallel low activity against prostaglandin synthesis in the rat stomach. After the characterization of the COX-2 gene, these three drugs were each found preferentially to inhibit COX-2 rather than COX-1, with a variation in their COX-2/COX-1 ratios of between 0.1 and 0.01 depending on the test system used. Ratios obtained by the human whole blood assay, which measures inhibition of COX-1 in platelets and COX-2 in mononuclear cells stimulated with LPS, are now generally accepted as the best reflection of the inhibitory activity of the drugs in humans (Table 1).

Meloxicam, which has a selectivity towards COX-2 of between 3- and 10-fold in the human whole blood assay and of 100-fold on human recombinant enzymes, is marketed around the world for use in rheumatoid arthritis and osteoarthritis[66]. In double-blind trials in many thousands of patients with osteoarthritis and rheumatoid arthritis, meloxicam in doses of 7.5 or 15 mg once daily compared in efficacy with standard NSAIDs such as naproxen 750–1000 mg, piroxicam 20 mg and diclofenac 100 mg. Both doses of meloxicam produced significantly fewer gastrointestinal adverse effects than the standard NSAIDs ($P<0.05$). Discontinuation of treatment due to gastrointestinal side effects was also significantly less frequent with meloxicam. PUBs occurred in fewer meloxicam-treated patients than in patients treated with piroxicam, diclofenac or naproxen. The frequency of adverse events with meloxicam (Figure 2) was significantly less at $P<0.05$ when compared to piroxicam and naproxen[67,68]. Clinical studies with meloxicam have been reviewed recently[69].

Etodolac is marketed in Europe and North America for the treatment of osteoarthritis and rheumatoid arthritis. It has an 11-fold selectivity for COX-2 over COX-1 when tested on recombinant human enzymes and about 5-fold selectivity in human whole blood[70]. In healthy human volunteers, etodolac twice daily did not suppress gastric mucosal prostaglandin production and caused less

Table 1 COX-2/COX-1 ratios of NSAIDs in the human whole blood assay

Drug	Patrignani et al. 1996[103]	Glaser et al. 1995[70]	Brideau et al. 1996[104], Prasit et al. 1997[105]	Warner et al. 1997[106]
Ketoprofen	1.7	–	50.0	2.0
Flurbiprofen	1.0	1.2	14.3	100.0
Indomethacin	0.5	2.5	3.3	33.0
Piroxicam	0.3	0.2	12.5	2.0
Naproxen	1.7	0.5	10.0	100.0
Ibuprofen	2.0	5.0	5.0	10.0
Diclofenac	–	0.3	0.5	0.33
Etodolac	–	0.12	0.20	0.19
Nimesulide	0.06	–	–	0.15
Meloxicam	0.09	–	0.33	0.20
Celecoxib	–	–	–	0.10
NS-398	0.006	0.006	0.10	0.24
SC-58125	0.007	<0.01	<<0.08	0.004
L-745,337	0.004	<<0.09	<<0.33	<0.1

Figure 2 Chemical structures of some selective COX-2 inhibitors

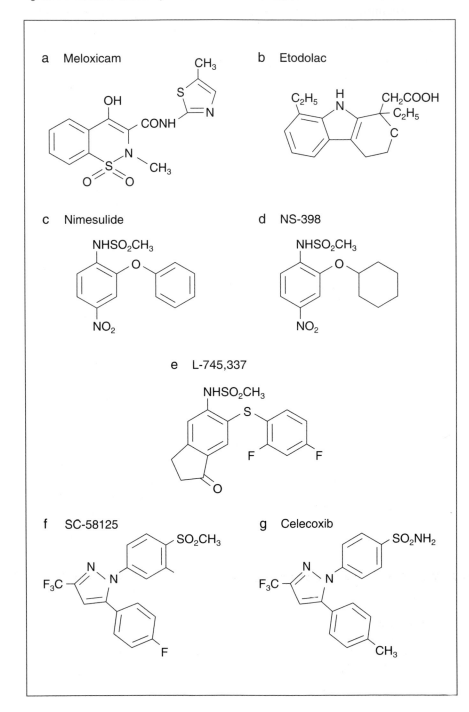

gastric damage than naproxen[71]. Patients with osteoarthritis or rheumatoid arthritis obtained relief from symptoms with etodolac equal to that of other commonly used NSAIDs (Figure 2) but with a lower incidence of serious gastrointestinal toxicity[72].

Nimesulide is currently sold in several European countries and in South America for the relief of pain associated with inflammatory conditions. It is a preferential inhibitor of COX-2 with about 5-fold greater potency against this enzyme than against COX-1 in the human whole blood assay (Table 1). In limited clinical trials for its use in acute and chronic inflammation in patients, it was more effective than placebo or had anti-inflammatory activity comparable to that of established NSAIDs[73–75]. Interestingly, nimesulide seems safe to use in aspirin-sensitive asthmatics. Several recent studies in NSAID-intolerant asthmatic patients demonstrated that therapeutic doses of nimesulide did not induce asthmatic attacks while high doses of 400 mg only precipitated mild asthma in 10% of patients[76]. A disadvantage of nimesulide (Figure 2) may be the need for dosing more than once a day because of its relatively short half life. This short half life is associated with high peak plasma concentrations which may take the drug levels into the inhibitory range for COX-1 (see Pairet, this volume). Certainly, the latest epidemiological study[77], which identified 1505 patients with upper gastrointestinal tract bleeding, shows nimesulide to have a similar relative risk to that of naproxen (4.4 times control) and more than diclofenac (2.7 times control). As with other NSAIDs, nimesulide is used in different dosages and when these are separated, the higher doses give a much higher relative risk.

Selective COX-2 Inhibitors in Clinical Development

The discovery of the COX-2 gene stimulated several laboratories to develop highly selective inhibitors of this enzyme. Needleman and his group at Monsanto/Searle have made inhibitors which are some 1000-fold more potent against COX-2 than against COX-1 in enzyme assays[78]. One of these, SC-58635 (celecoxib), is an effective analgesic for moderate to severe pain following tooth extraction[79]. Celecoxib (Figure 2) given for 7 days to human volunteers provided no evidence of gastric damage[80]. It is currently in Phase III clinical trials in arthritic patients[78]. Interestingly, in the whole blood assay, celecoxib is only 10-fold more active against COX-2 than COX-1 (Table 1).

A similar highly selective COX-2 inhibitor from Merck-Frosst, MK-966 (Vioxx), which is an analogue of an earlier Merck compound L-745,337 (Figure 2), is currently undergoing Phase III clinical trials[81]. In Phase I studies, a single dose of 250 mg daily for 7 days (which is ten times the anti-inflammatory dose) produced no adverse effects on the stomach mucosa, as evidenced by gastroscopy[82]. After a single dose of 1 g, there was no evidence of COX-1 inhibition in platelets, but activity of COX-2 in LPS-stimulated monocytes ex vivo was reduced. For post-operative dental pain, MK-966 at 25 mg per dose demonstrated analgesic activity equal to that of ibuprofen, and provided relief from symptoms in a 6-week study of osteoarthritis[83].

FUTURE THERAPEUTIC USES FOR SELECTIVE COX-2 INHIBITORS

Premature Labour

Prostaglandins induce uterine contractions during labour. NSAIDs such as indomethacin will delay premature labour by inhibiting the production of prostaglandins, but will at the same time cause early closure of the ductus arteriosus and reduce urine production by the foetal kidneys[84]. The delay in the birth process is most likely due to inhibition of COX-2 since mRNA for COX-2 increases substantially in the amnion and placenta immediately before and after the start of labour[85], whereas the side effects on the foetus are due to inhibition of COX-1. One cause of pre-term labour could be an intra-uterine infection resulting in release of endogenous factors that increase prostaglandin production by upregulating COX-2[54]. Nimesulide reduces prostaglandin synthesis in isolated foetal membranes and has been used successfully for a prolonged period to delay premature labour without manifesting the side effects of indomethacin on the foetus[84].

Colon Cancer

Epidemiological studies have established a strong link between ingestion of aspirin and a reduced risk of developing colon cancer[86,87]. Sulindac also caused reduction of prostaglandin synthesis and regression of adenomatous polyps in 11 out of 15 patients with familial adenomatous polyposis (FAP), a condition in which many colorectal polyps develop spontaneously with eventual progression to tumours[88-90]. This indication that COX activity is involved in the process leading to colon cancer is supported by the demonstration that COX-2 and not COX-1 is highly expressed in human and animal colon cancer cells as well as in human colorectal adenocarcinomas[35,36]. Further support for the close connection between COX-2 and colon cancer has come from studies in the mutant *Apc* mouse, which is a model of FAP in humans. The spontaneous development of intestinal polyposis in these mice was strongly reduced either by deletion of the COX-2 gene or by treatment with a highly selective COX-2 inhibitor[91-93]. Nimesulide also reduced the number and size of intestinal polyps in *Min* mice[94]. The development of azoxymethane-induced colon tumours over a year was inhibited in celecoxib-fed rats[95]. Thus, it is highly likely that COX-2 inhibitors could be used prophylactically to prevent colon cancer in genetically susceptible individuals, without causing gastrointestinal damage themselves.

Alzheimer's Disease

The connection between COX and Alzheimer's disease has been based entirely on epidemiology largely due to the lack of an animal model of the disease. A number of studies have shown a significantly reduced odds ratio for Alzheimer's disease in those taking NSAIDs as anti-inflammatory therapy[96-98]. The Baltimore Longitudinal Study of Aging, with 1686 participants, reported in 1997 that the risk of developing Alzheimer's disease is reduced among users of NSAIDs, especially those who have taken the medications for two years or more[99]. No decreased risk was evident with acetaminophen or aspirin use. However, aspirin was probably taken in a dose too low to have an anti-inflammatory effect. The protective effect of NSAIDs is consistent with evidence of inflammatory activity in the pathophysiology of Alzheimer's disease[100,101]. However, the content of COX-2 in brain tissue of Alzheimer's disease patients was lower than normal[102], which may reflect the large loss of neuronal tissue in the late stages of the disease. Chronic treatment with selective COX-2 inhibitors may therefore slow the progress of Alzheimer's disease without damaging the stomach mucosa[99].

CONCLUSIONS

The identification of selective inhibitors of COX-2 will clearly provide important advances in the therapy of inflammation. Conventional NSAIDs lead to gastrointestinal side effects, which include ulceration of the stomach, sometimes with subsequent perforation, and deaths estimated at several thousand a year in the USA alone[59]. The evidence is strong, both from animal tests and from the clinic that the selective COX-2 inhibitors will have greatly reduced side effects.

All the results so far published (and many reported at meetings, but yet to be published in the literature), support the hypothesis that the unwanted side effects of NSAIDs are due to their ability to inhibit COX-1 whilst their anti-inflammatory (therapeutic effects) are due to inhibition of COX-2. This concept is now set in stone. Thus, selective COX-2 inhibitors will provide an important advance in anti-inflammatory therapy. They are unlikely to be more potent anti-inflammatory agents than the conventional NSAIDs, but they will have the tremendous advantage of being safer and better tolerated. Already, the clinical results with meloxicam show this improved safety and tolerability, even though it retains some activity against COX-1.

In addition to their beneficial actions in inflammatory diseases, these drugs may be useful in the future for the prevention of colon cancer, Alzheimer's disease or premature labour.

REFERENCES

1. Whitehouse MW, Haslam JM. Ability of some antirheumatic drugs to uncouple oxidative phosphorylation. *Nature*. 1962;196:1323–4.
2. Hines WJW, Smith MJH. Inhibition of dehydrogenases by salicylate. *Nature*. 1964;201:192.
3. Smith MJH, Bryant C, Hines WJW. Reversal by nicotinamide adenine dinucleotide of the inhibitory action of salicylate on mitochondrial malate dehydrogenase. *Nature*. 1964;202:96–7.
4. Gould BJ, Smith MJH. Salicylate and aminotransferases. *J Pharm Pharmacol*. 1965;17:83–8.
5. Gould BJ, Smith MJH. Inhibition of rat brain glutamate decarboxylase activity by salicylate in vitro. *J Pharm Pharmacol*. 1965;17:15–8.

6. Weiss WP, Campbell PL, Diebler GE, Sokoloff L. Effects of salicylate on amino acid incorporation into protein. *J Pharmacol Exp Ther*. 1962;136:366–71.

7. Vane JR. The use of isolated organs for detecting active substances in the circulating blood. *Br J Pharmacol Chemother*. 1964;23:360–73.

8. Piper PJ, Vane JR. The release of prostaglandins during anaphylaxis in guinea-pig isolated lungs. In: Mantegazza P, Horton EW, editors. *Prostaglandins, Peptides and Amines*. London/New York: Academic Press; 1969:15–19.

9. Hamberg M, Svensson J, Samuelsson B. Thromboxanes: a new group of biologically active compounds derived from prostaglandin endoperoxides. *Proc Natl Acad Sci USA*. 1975;72:2994–8.

10. Palmer MA, Piper PJ, Vane JR. The release of RCS from chopped lung and its antagonism by anti-inflammatory drugs. *Br J Pharmacol*. 1970;40:581P.

11. Vane JR. Inhibition of prostaglandin synthesis as a mechanism of action for aspirin-like drugs. *Nat New Biol*. 1971;231:232–5.

12. Smith JH, Willis AL. Aspirin selectively inhibits prostaglandin production in human platelets. *Nature*. 1971;231:235–7.

13. Ferreira SH, Moncada S, Vane JR. Indomethacin and aspirin abolish prostaglandin release from spleen. *Nature*. 1971;231:237–9.

14. Flower RJ, Vane JR. Inhibition of prostaglandin biosynthesis. *Biochem Pharmacol*. 1974;23:1439–50.

15. Higgs GA, Moncada S, Vane JR. Eicosanoids in inflammation. *Ann Clin Res*. 1984;16:287–99.

16. Vane JR, Botting RM. The mode of action of anti-inflammatory drugs. *Postgrad Med J*. 1990;66(suppl 4):S2–S17.

17. Hemler M, Lands WEM, Smith WL. Purification of the cyclo-oxygenase that forms prostaglandins. Demonstration of the two forms of iron in the holoenzyme. *J Biol Chem*. 1976;251:5575–9.

18. DeWitt DL, Smith WL. Primary structure of prostaglandin G/H synthase from sheep vesicular gland determined from the complementary DNA sequence. *Proc Natl Acad Sci USA*. 1988;85:1412–6.

19. Merlie JP, Fagan D, Mudd J, Needleman P. Isolation and characterization of the complementary DNA for sheep seminal vesicle prostaglandin endoperoxide synthase (cyclooxygenase). *J Biol Chem*. 1988;263:3550–3.

20. Yokoyama C, Takai T, Tanabe T. Primary structure of sheep prostaglandin endoperoxide synthase deduced from cDNA sequence. *FEBS Lett*. 1988;231:347–51.

21. Picot D, Loll PJ, Garavito RM. The X-ray crystal structure of the membrane protein prostaglandin H_2 synthase-1. *Nature*. 1994;367:243–9.

22. Roth GJ, Stanford N, Majerus PW. Acetylation of prostaglandin synthetase by aspirin. *Proc Natl Acad Sci USA*. 1975;72:3073–6.

23. Luong C, Miller A, Barnett J, Chow J, Ramesha C, Browner MF. Flexibility of the NSAID binding site in the structure of human cyclooxygenase-2. *Nat Struct Biol*. 1996;3:927–33.

24. Moncada S, Gryglewski R, Bunting S, Vane JR. An enzyme isolated from arteries transforms prostaglandin endoperoxides to an unstable substance that inhibits platelet aggregation. *Nature*. 1976;263:663–5.

25. Whittle BJR, Higgs GA, Eakins KE, Moncada S, Vane JR. Selective inhibition of prostaglandin production in inflammatory exudates and gastric mucosa. *Nature*. 1980;284:271–3.

26. Xie W, Robertson DL, Simmons DL. Mitogen-inducible prostaglandin G/H synthase: a new target for nonsteroidal antiinflammatory drugs. *Drug Devel Res*. 1992;25:249–65.

27. Fu J-Y, Masferrer JL, Seibert K, Raz A, Needleman P. The induction and suppression of prostaglandin H$_2$ synthase (cyclooxygenase) in human monocytes. *J Biol Chem.* 1990;265:16737–40.

28. Masferrer JL, Zweifel BS, Seibert K, Needleman P. Selective regulation of cellular cyclooxygenase by dexamethasone and endotoxin in mice. *J Clin Invest.* 1990;86:1375–9.

29. Xie W, Chipman JG, Robertson DL, Erikson RL, Simmons DL. Expression of a mitogen-responsive gene encoding prostaglandin synthase is regulated by mRNA splicing. *Proc Natl Acad Sci USA.* 1991;88:2692–6.

30. O'Banion MK, Sadowski HB, Winn V, Young DA. A serum- and glucocorticoid-regulated 4-kilobase mRNA encodes a cyclooxygenase-related protein. *J Biol Chem.* 1991;266:23261–7.

31. Kujubu DA, Fletcher BS, Varnum BC, Lim RW, Herschman HR. TIS10, a phorbol ester tumor promoter-inducible mRNA from Swiss 3T3 cells, encodes a novel prostaglandin synthase/cyclooxygenase homologue. *J Biol Chem.* 1991;266:12866–72.

32. Sirois J, Richards JS. Purification and characterisation of a novel, distinct isoform of prostaglandin endoperoxide synthase induced by human chorionic gonadotropin in granulosa cells of rat preovulatory follicles. *J Biol Chem.* 1992;267:6382–8.

33. Whittle BJR, Vane JR. Prostanoids as regulators of gastrointestinal function. In: Johnston LR, editor. *Physiology of the Gastrointestinal Tract.* Vol I, 2nd edn. New York: Raven Press; 1987:143–80.

34. Kargman S, Charleson S, Cartwright M, Frank J, Riendeau D, Mancini J et al. Characterization of prostaglandin G/H synthase 1 and 2 in rat, dog, monkey and human gastrointestinal tracts. *Gastroenterology.* 1996;111:445–54.

35. Kutchera W, Jones DA, Matsunami N, Groden J, McIntyre TM, Zimmerman GA et al. Prostaglandin H synthase 2 is expressed abnormally in human colon cancer: Evidence for a transcriptional effect. *Proc Natl Acad Sci USA.* 1996;93:4816–20.

36. Gustafson-Svärd C, Lilja I, Hallböök O, Sjödahl R. Cyclooxygenase-1 and cyclooxygenase-2 gene expression in human colorectal adenocarcinomas and in azoxymethane induced colonic tumours in rats. *Gut.* 1996;38:79–84.

37. Langenbach R, Morham SG, Tiano HF, Loftin CD, Ghanayem BI, Chulada PC et al. Prostaglandin synthase 1 gene disruption in mice reduces arachidonic acid-induced inflammation and indomethacin-induced gastric ulceration. *Cell.* 1995;83:483–92.

38. Whittle BJR. Neuronal and endothelium-derived mediators in the modulation of the gastric microcirculation: integrity in the balance. *Br J Pharmacol.* 1993;110:3–17.

39. Harris RC, McKanna JA, Akai Y, Jacobson HR, Dubois RN, Breyer MD. Cyclooxygenase-2 is associated with the macula densa of rat kidney and increases with salt restriction. *J Clin Invest.* 1994;94:2504–10.

40. Morham SG, Langenbach R, Loftin CD, Tiano HF, Vouloumanos N, Jenette JC et al. Prostaglandin synthase 2 gene disruption causes renal pathology in the mouse. *Cell.* 1995;83:473–82.

41. Yamagata K, Andreasson KI, Kaufman WE, Barnes CA, Worley PF. Expression of a mitogen-inducible cyclooxygenase in brain neurons; regulation by synaptic activity and glucocorticoids. *Neuron.* 1993;11:371–86.

42. Breder CD, Dewitt D, Kraig RP. Characterization of inducible cyclooxygenase in rat brain. *J Comp Neurol.* 1995;355:296–315.

43. Breder CD, Saper CB. Expression of inducible cyclooxygenase mRNA in the mouse brain after systemic administration of bacterial lipopolysaccharide. *Brain Res.* 1996;713:64–9.

44. Cao C, Matsumura K, Yamagata K, Watanabe Y. Endothelial cells of the brain vasculature express cyclooxygenase-2 mRNA in response to systemic interleukin-1β: a possible site of prostaglandin synthesis responsible for fever. *Brain Res.* 1996;733:263–72.

45. Cao C, Matsumura K, Yamagata K, Watanabe Y. Induction by lipopolysaccharide of cyclooxygenase-2 mRNA in rat brain; its possible role in the febrile response. *Brain Res.* 1995;697:187–96.

46. Marcheselli VL, Bazan NG. Sustained induction of prostaglandin endoperoxide synthase-2 by seizures in hippocampus. *J Biol Chem.* 1996;271:24794–9.

47. Beiche F, Scheuerer S, Brune K, Geisslinger G, Goppelt-Struebe M. Up-regulation of cyclooxygenase-2 mRNA in the rat spinal cord following peripheral inflammation. *FEBS Lett.* 1996;390:165–9.

48. Futaki N, Yoshikawa K, Hamasaka Y, Arai I, Higuchi S, Iizuka H et al. NS-398, a novel non-steroidal anti-inflammatory drug with potent analgesic and antipyretic effects which causes minimal stomach lesions. *Gen Pharmacol.* 1993;24:105–10.

49. Bennett P, Slater D. COX-2 expression in labour. In: Vane J, Botting J, Botting R, editors. *Improved Non-steroid Anti-inflammatory Drugs. COX-2 Enzyme Inhibitors.* Lancaster: Kluwer Academic Publishers and London: William Harvey Press;1996:167–88.

50. Gibb W, Sun M. Localization of prostaglandin H synthase type 2 protein and mRNA in term human fetal membranes and decidua. *J Endocrinol.* 1996;150:497–503.

51. Trautman MS, Edwin SS, Collmer D, Dudley DJ, Simmons D, Mitchell MD. Prostaglandin H synthase-2 in human gestational tissues: Regulation in amnion. *Placenta.* 1996;17:239–45.

52. Toth P, Li X, Lei ZM, Rao CV. Expression of human chorionic gonadotropin (hCG)/luteinizing hormone receptors and regulation of the cyclooxygenase-1 gene by exogenous hCG in human fetal membranes. *J Clin Endocrinol Metab.* 1996;81:1283–8.

53. Zakar T, Hirst JJ, Milovic JE, Olson DM. Glucocorticoids stimulate the expression of prostaglandin endoperoxide H synthase-2 in amnion cells. *Endocrinology.* 1995;136:1610–9.

54. Spaziani EP, Lantz ME, Benoit RR, O'Brien WF. The induction of cyclooxygenase-2 (COX-2) in intact human amnion tissue by interleukin-4. *Prostaglandins.* 1996;51:215–23.

55. Chakraborty I, Das SK, Wang J, Dey SK. Developmental expression of the cyclo-oxygenase-1 and cyclo-oxygenase-2 genes in the peri-implantation mouse uterus and their differential regulation by the blastocyst and ovarian steroids. *J Mol Endocrinol.* 1996;16:107–22.

56. Dinchuck JE, Car BD, Focht RJ, Johnston JJ, Jaffee BD, Covington MB et al. Renal abnormalities and an altered inflammatory response in mice lacking cyclooxygenase II. *Nature.* 1995;378:406–9.

57. Henry D, Lim LL-Y, Garcia Rodriguez LA, Perez Gutthann S, Carson JL, Griffin M et al. Variability in risk of gastrointestinal complications with individual non-steroidal anti-inflammatory drugs: results of a collaborative meta-analysis. *Br Med J.* 1996; 312:1563–6.

58. Coles LS, Fries JF, Kraines RG, Roth SH. From experiment to experience: side effects of nonsteroidal anti-inflammatory drugs. *Am J Med.* 1983;74:820–8.

59. Fries J. Toward an understanding of NSAID-related adverse events: the contribution of longitudinal data. *Scand J Rheumatol.* 1996;25(suppl 102):3–8.

60. Mitchell JA, Akarasereenont P, Thiemermann C, Flower RJ, Vane JR. Selectivity of non-steroidal antiinflammatory drugs as inhibitors of constitutive and inducible cyclooxygenase. *Proc Natl Acad Sci USA.* 1993;90;11693–7.

61. Meade EA, Smith WL, DeWitt DL. Differential inhibition of prostaglandin endoperoxide synthase (cyclooxygenase) isozymes by aspirin and other non-steroidal anti-inflammatory drugs. *J Biol Chem.* 1993;268:6610–4.

62. Lanza FL. A review of gastric ulcer and gastroduodenal injury in normal volunteers receiving aspirin and other non-steroidal anti-inflammatory drugs. *Scand J Gastroenterol.* 1989;24(suppl 163):24–31.

63. Akarasereenont P, Mitchell JA, Thiemermann C, Vane JR. Relative potency of nonsteroid anti-inflammatory drugs as inhibitors of cyclooxygenase-1 or cyclooxygenase-2. *Br J Pharmacol*. 1994;112(suppl):183P.

64. Garcia Rodriguez LA, Jick H. Risk of upper gastrointestinal bleeding and perforation associated with individual non-steroidal anti-inflammatory drugs. *Lancet*. 1994;343:769–72.

65. Vane JR, Botting RM. New insights into the mode of action of anti-inflammatory drugs. *Inflamm Res*. 1995;44:1–10.

66. Churchill L, Graham AG, Shih C-K, Pauletti D, Farina PR, Grob PM. Selective inhibition of human cyclo-oxygenase-2 by meloxicam. *Inflammopharmacology*. 1996;4:125–35.

67. Barner A. Review of clinical trials and benefit/risk ratio of meloxicam. *Scand J Rheumatol*. 1996;25(suppl 102):29–37.

68. Distel M, Mueller C, Bluhmki E, Fries J. Safety of meloxicam: a global analysis of clinical trials. *Br J Rheumatol*. 1996;35(suppl 1):68–77.

69. Degner F, Turck D, Pairet M. Pharmacological, pharmacokinetic and clinical profile of meloxicam. *Drugs Today*. 1997;33:739–58.

70. Glaser K, Sung M-L, O'Neill K, Belfast M, Hartman D, Carlson R et al. Etodolac selectively inhibits human prostaglandin G/H synthase 2 (PGHS-2) versus human PGHS-1. *Eur J Pharmacol*. 1995;281:107–11.

71. Laine L, Sloane R, Ferretti M, Cominelli F. A randomised double-blind comparison of placebo, etodolac and naproxen on gastrointestinal injury and prostaglandin production. *Gastrointest Endosc*. 1995;42:428–33.

72. Cummings DM, Amadio P Jr. A review of selected newer nonsteroidal anti-inflammatory drugs. *Am Fam Physician*. 1994;49:1197–202.

73. Weissenbach R. Clinical trials with nimesulide, a new non-steroid anti-inflammatory agent, in rheumatic pathology. *J Int Med Res*. 1981;13:237–45.

74. Pais JM, Rosteito FM. Nimesulide in the short-term treatment of the inflammatory process of dental tissues: a double-blind controlled trial against oxyphenbutazone. *J Int Med Res*. 1983;11:149–54.

75. Emami Nouri E. Nimesulide for treatment of acute inflammation of the upper respiratory tract. *Clin Ther*. 1984;6:142–50.

76. Senna GE, Passalacqua G, Andri G, Dama AR, Albano M, Fregonese L et al. Nimesulide in the treatment of patients intolerant of aspirin and other NSAIDs. *Drug Safety*. 1996;14:94–103.

77. Garcia Rodriguez LA, Cattaruzzi C, Troncom MG, Agostinis L. Risk of hospitalization for upper gastrointestinal tract bleeding associated with ketorolac, other nonsteroidal anti-inflammatory drugs, calcium antagonists, and other antihypertensive drugs. *Arch Intern Med*. 1998;158:33–39.

78. Isakson P, Zweifel B, Masferrer J, Koboldt C, Seibert K, Hubbard R et al. Specific COX-2 inhibitors: from bench to bedside. In: Vane J, Botting J, editors. *Selective COX-2 Inhibitors. Pharmacology, Clinical Effects and Therapeutic Potential*. London: Kluwer Academic Publishers and William Harvey Press; 1998:1–17.

79. Hubbard RC, Mehlisch DR, Jasper DR, Nugent MJ, Yu S, Isakson PC. SC-58635, a highly selective inhibitor of COX-2, is an effective analgesic in an acute post-surgical pain model. *J Invest Med*. 1996;44:293A.

80. Lanza FL, Rack MF, Callison DA, Hubbard RC, Yu SS, Talwalker S et al. A pilot endoscopic study of the gastroduodenal effects of SC-58635, a novel COX-2 selective inhibitor. *Gastroenterology*. 1997;112:A194.

81. Ford-Hutchinson AW. New highly selective COX-2 inhibitors. In: Vane J, Botting J, editors. *Selective COX-2 Inhibitors. Pharmacology, Clinical Effects and Therapeutic Potential*. London: Kluwer Academic Publishers and William Harvey Press; 1998:117–25.

82. Lanza F, Simon T, Quan H, Bolognese J, Rack MF, Hoover M et al. Selective inhibition of cyclooxygenase-2 (COX-2) with MK-0966 (250 mg q.d.) is associated with less gastro-duodenal damage than aspirin (ASA) 650 mg q.i.d. or ibuprofen (IBU) 800 mg t.i.d. *Gastroenterology.* 1997;112:A194.

83. Ehrich E, Mehlisch D, Perkins S, Brown P, Wittreich J, Lipschutz K et al. Efficacy of MK-966, a highly selective inhibitor of COX-2, in the treatment of postoperative dental pain. *Arthritis Rheum.* 1996;39(suppl 9):S81.

84. Sawdy R, Slater D, Fisk N, Edmonds DK, Bennett P. Use of a cyclo-oxygenase type-2-selective non-steroidal anti-inflammatory agent to prevent preterm delivery. *Lancet.* 1997;350:265–6.

85. Gibb W, Sun M. Localization of prostaglandin H synthase type 2 protein and mRNA in term human fetal membranes and decidua. *J Endocrinol.* 1996;150:497–503.

86. Thun MJ, Namboodiri MM, Heath CWJ. Aspirin use and reduced risk of fatal colon cancer. *N Engl J Med.* 1991;325:1593–6.

87. Luk GD. Prevention of gastrointestinal cancer – the potential role of NSAIDs in colorectal cancer. *Schweiz Med Wochenschr.* 1996;126:801–12.

88. Nugent KP, Spigelman AD, Phillips RKS. Tissue prostaglandin levels in familial adenomatous polyposis patients treated with sulindac. *Dis Colon Rectum.* 1996;39:659–62.

89. Giardiello FM, Hamilton SR, Krush AJ, Piantadosi S, Hyland LM, Celano P et al. Treatment of colonic and rectal adenomas with sulindac in familial adenomatous polyposis. *N Engl J Med.* 1993;328:1313–6.

90. Matsuhashi N, Nakajima A, Fukushima Y, Yazaki Y, Oka T. Effects of sulindac on sporadic colorectal adenomatous polyps. *Gut.* 1997;40:344–9.

91. Eberhart CE, Coffey RJ, Radhika A, Giardiello FM, Ferrenbach S, DuBois RN. Up-regulation of cyclooxygenase 2 gene expression in human colorectal adenomas and adenocarcinomas. *Gastroenterology.* 1994;104:1183–8.

92. Sheng H, Shao J, Kirkland SC, Isakson P, Coffey RJ, Morrow J et al. Inhibition of human colon cancer cell growth by selective inhibition of cyclooxygenase-2. *J Clin Invest.* 1997;99:2254–9.

93. Oshima M, Dinchuk JE, Kargman SL, Oshima H, Hancock B, Kwong E et al. Suppression of intestinal polyposis in $Apc^{\Delta716}$ knockout mice by inhibition of cyclooxygenase 2 (COX-2). *Cell.* 1996;87:803–9.

94. Nakatsugi S, Fukutake M, Takahashi M, Fukuda K, Isoi T, Taniguchi Y et al. Suppression of intestinal polyp development by nimesulide, a selective cyclooxygenase-2 inhibitor, in Min mice. *Jpn J Cancer Res.* 1997;88:1117–20.

95. Kawamori T, Rao CV, Seibert K, Reddy BS. Chemopreventive activity of celecoxib a specific cyclooxygenase-2 inhibitor, against colon carcinogenesis. *Cancer Res.* 1998;58:409–12.

96. Cochran FR, Vitek MP. Neuroinflammatory mechanisms in Alzheimer's disease: new opportunities for drug discovery. *Expert Opin Invest Drugs.* 1996;5:449–55.

97. Breitner JCS. The role of anti-inflammatory drugs in the prevention and treatment of Alzheimer's disease. *Annu Rev Med.* 1996;47:401–11.

98. McGeer PL, McGeer EG. The inflammatory response system of brain: implications for therapy of Alzheimer and other neurodegenerative diseases. *Brain Res Rev.* 1995;21:195–218.

99. Stewart WF, Kawas C, Corrada M, Metter EJ. Risk of Alzheimer's disease and duration of NSAID use. *Neurology.* 1997;48:626–32.

100. Hampel H, Muller N. Inflammatory and immunological mechanisms in Alzheimer's disease. *Drug News Perspect.* 1995;8:599–608.

101. Yan SD, Zhu H, Fu J, Yan SF, Roher A, Tourtellotte WW et al. Amyloid-β peptide-receptor for advanced glycation endproduct interaction elicits neuronal expression of macrophage-colony stimulating factor: a proinflammatory pathway in Alzheimer disease. *Proc Natl Acad Sci USA.* 1997;94:5296–301.

102. Chang JW, Coleman PD, O'Banion MK. Prostaglandin G/H synthase-2 (cyclooxygenase-2) mRNA expression is decreased in Alzheimer's disease. *Neurobiol Aging.* 1996;17:801–8.

103. Partrignani P, Panara MR, Santini G, Sciulli MG, Padovano R, Cipollone F. Differential inhibition of cyclooxygenase activity of prostaglandin endoperoxide synthase isozymes in vitro and ex vivo in man. *Prostaglandins Leukot Essent Fatty Acids.* 1996;55(suppl 1):P115.

104. Brideau C, Kargman S, Liu S, Dallob AL, Ehrich FW, Rodger IW et al. A human whole blood assay for clinical evaluation of biochemical efficacy of cyclooxygenase inhibitors. *Inflamm Res.* 1996;45:68–74.

105. Prasit P. New highly selective COX-2 inhibitors. William Harvey Research Conference. Selective COX-2 Inhibitors. Phuket, Sept 18–19, 1997.

106. Warner T, Vojnovic I. Unpublished observations. 1997.

2

Tests for cyclooxygenase-1 and -2 inhibition

M. PAIRET AND J. VAN RYN

The anti-inflammatory effects of non-steroidal anti-inflammatory drugs (NSAIDs) are thought to occur through a mechanism different from that of the adverse effects seen with these compounds. Side effects such as disruption of gastric cytoprotection, renal function and inhibition of platelet function appear to result from the inhibition of cyclooxygenase (COX)-1[1]. COX-1 is a constitutive isoenzyme, or 'housekeeping' enzyme, which is found under physiological conditions in most tissues[2]. In contrast, COX-2 is not usually present in cells under basal conditions, but its expression is induced during inflammatory processes[3-5]. Thus, it appears that the relevant target for the anti-inflammatory effects of NSAIDs is COX-2 inhibition, whereas the gastric and renal side effects are due to COX-1 inhibition[1-3].

To compare the inhibition of COX-1 and COX-2 by various NSAIDs, numerous assays have been developed[6]. The results from these assays are used to calculate a measure of COX-2 selectivity, and then NSAIDs are compared to each other by ranking their COX-2 selectivity. However, the many test systems developed have resulted in different COX-1/COX-2 ratios, sometimes for the same drug, and thus to confusing comparisons.

By providing a critical analysis of the in vitro assays available and demonstrating the problems with interpretation of the results, COX-1 and COX-2 selectivity of various NSAIDs can be assessed. In addition, the in vivo relevance of in vitro findings will be discussed, including pharmacokinetic properties of the NSAIDs and results from human pharmacological studies.

COMPARISON OF NSAIDS USING SELECTIVITY RATIOS

The commonly used in vitro assays for investigating the COX-1 and COX-2 selectivity of NSAIDs can be divided into three groups. The first consists of assays using animal enzymes, animal cells or cell lines[7–11]. These were the first tests to be developed and are historical in nature. The second type of assay uses human recombinant enzymes, human cell lines or human blood cells (mainly platelets and monocytes)[12–23]. These are the standard tests performed today. The third group consists of newly developed models using human cells that are targets for the anti-inflammatory and side effects of NSAIDs. These targets include human gastric mucosal cells[24], chondrocytes[25] and synoviocytes[26,27].

Several aspects should be considered when comparing the relative selectivity of NSAIDs on COX inhibition from these different test systems. Generally speaking, it should be obvious that comparison of selectivity ratios among NSAIDs is only valid when all the inhibitors are tested in the same assay system. Comparing different compounds with results obtained from different assays can become confusing[28,29].

Thus, there are several important factors to consider when 'pooling' results obtained from different sources to compare COX-2 selectivity of NSAIDs. The COX enzymes used in these assays can be of animal or human origin, they can be native or recombinant, and they can be used either as purified enzymes, microsomal preparations or whole cell assays. In addition, prostaglandin synthesis can be measured either from endogenously released arachidonic acid or from exogenously added arachidonic acid. In assays using recombinant COX-1 and COX-2 enzymes, the expression system used for gene replication also varies. Not all assay systems use a COX-2 inducing agent. For instance, cells that are transfected with recombinant enzymes express this enzyme constitutively. However, in other cells COX-2 has to be induced. COX-2 is usually induced with either lipopolysaccharide (LPS) or cytokines, such as interleukin-1 (IL-1) or tumour necrosis factor. In addition, the duration of the incubation with the drug being tested and with the inducing agent differs between laboratories. This is particularly important, since the inhibition of COX-2 is time-dependent. Also important is the protein concentration in the assay, since NSAIDs are known to bind avidly to plasma proteins.

While the results of most assays are expressed as selectivity ratios, the criteria used to generate these ratios can also vary. Selectivity ratios are obtained by dividing the IC_{50} value for inhibition of COX-1 by the IC_{50} value for the inhibition of COX-2 (the higher the ratio, the greater the COX-2 selectivity), or conversely (the lower the ratio, the greater the COX-1 selectivity). However, the limits of such calculations need to be considered. Theoretically, such ratios may only be calculated when the concentration–response curves (linear portion) are parallel (Figure 1a). In practice, this criterion is not always fulfilled (Figure 1b).

Selectivity ratios should also be available from several representative models before the degree of COX-2 inhibition is considered. The importance of each test system should also be taken into account. Results obtained with human whole cells may be more representative of in vivo efficacy than results obtained using animal enzymes in an artificial situation. This can be demonstrated by results obtained with nabumetone, where a preferential inhibition of COX-2 was obtained using mouse recombinant enzymes[11]. However, this could not be

Figure I Concentration–response curves for COX-I and COX-2 inhibition and calculation of selectivity ratios

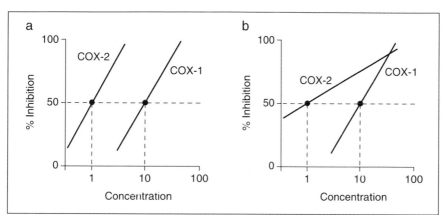

confirmed using human recombinant enzymes[16,17] or a human whole blood assay[18,19] in vitro, and could also not be confirmed in vivo[30].

CLINICAL RELEVANCE OF COX-2 SELECTIVITY

The objective of a study should be the first consideration when choosing an assay system. Purified enzymes are the ideal targets if the aim is to investigate the interaction between a drug and the active site of the enzyme at the molecular level. Human cell lines which constitutively express either COX-1 or COX-2, or human recombinant enzymes in a microsomal assay, allow a high throughput, and are best suited for screening or for structure–activity relationship studies. However, to investigate the clinical relevance of selective COX-2 inhibition, the following considerations should determine the choice of the assay used.

Native human enzymes that are present in whole cells should be used and the cells used in this assay should be target cells for the anti-inflammatory and side effects of NSAIDs. COX-2 should be induced, since this more closely simulates an inflammatory process. Prostaglandin synthesis should result from the utilization of endogenously released arachidonic acid, rather than from exogenously added substrate. In addition, protein concentration in the assay medium should mimic plasma protein concentration so that NSAID binding to proteins is taken into account. The systems most commonly used when considering clinical relevance are human recombinant enzymes in whole cells and the human whole blood assay. These systems constitute the best compromise to date between the characteristics of an ideal model and the practical feasibility of performing an assay.

When establishing the clinical relevance of an assay, it is tempting to compare the IC_{50} values obtained in vitro to concentrations of a drug in human plasma obtained ex vivo. However, this should only be done if drug binding to plasma proteins has been taken into account in the in vitro assay, which is usually not the case. One assay that allows for protein binding is the human whole blood assay, and the plasma proteins in whole blood may better represent in vivo interactions in the presence of NSAIDs.

Despite these many considerations, COX-2 selectivity in vitro is still best expressed using selectivity ratios. However, at most these ratios should be considered as showing trends. They are not sufficient to predict the level of inhibition of COX-1 and COX-2 in vivo after administration of a particular dose. In addition, data of COX-1 and COX-2 inhibition obtained in vivo (or ex vivo) should always have priority over in vitro data.

HUMAN WHOLE BLOOD ASSAY

Whole human clotting blood is used to test for inhibition of COX-1 activity, and whole blood stimulated by LPS is used to test for inhibition of COX-2 activity in this assay. There are many advantages to using this assay. Intact human cells are used that are target cells for the anti-inflammatory effects (monocytes) and side effects (platelets) of NSAIDs in the presence of plasma proteins. Whole blood used for both assays is taken from the same volunteer (or patient) at the same time, thereby allowing a direct comparison of the results. The main drawback is that different incubation times are used for COX-1 and COX-2, since COX-2 has to be induced.

The effects of various NSAIDs using the human whole blood assay are summarized in Table 1. Standard NSAIDs are approximately equally effective in inhibiting both isoenzymes. Diclofenac has the most favourable profile of the

Table 1 COX-2 selectivity expressed as the IC_{50} of COX-1 /IC_{50} of COX-2 ratio for various NSAIDs in a human whole blood assay

	Glaser et al.[15]	Patrigniani et al.[18]	Brideau et al.[20], Prasit[21]	Pairet et al.[22]	Warner[23]
Ketoprofen	–	0.6	0.02	–	–
Flurbiprofen	0.8	1.0	0.07	–	0.01
Indomethacin	0.4	1.9	0.3	1.2	0.02
Piroxicam	4.5	3.1	0.08	0.9	0.5
Naproxen	2.0	0.6	0.1	–	0.006
Ibuprofen	0.2	0.5	0.2	–	0.1
6-MNA	–	1.5	0.3	–	–
Diclofenac	3.0	–	2.0	3.5	2.8
Etodolac	8.1	–	5.0	–	5.3
Nimesulide	–	17.7	–	–	6.5
Meloxicam	–	11.2	3.0	13.1	5.0
SC-58635	–	–	–	34.7	9.6
Flosulide	–	–	40.0	–	–
DuP-697	–	–	20.0	–	–
NS-398	155.0	168.0	10.0	–	4.1
SC-58125	>100	143.3	>13	37.2	–
L-745,337	>11	146.0	>3	–	–

standard NSAIDs. Compounds such as etodolac, nimesulide and meloxicam inhibit COX-2 preferentially (ratio 3 to 30), while flosulide, DuP-697, NS-398, L-745,337 and SC-58125 are selective for COX-2.

A comparison of results obtained with the whole blood assay and with the human recombinant enzyme assay in whole cells is shown in Figure 2. The bars indicate the range of ratios obtained with the same model by different laboratories. Although a parallel trend is evident, the range of selectivity ratios is wider when recombinant enzymes are used than with the whole blood assay.

IN VIVO RELEVANCE OF IN VITRO RESULTS

The in vivo relevance of in vitro results of COX-2 selectivity should be considered carefully. The assay system in which the NSAID selectivity ratio was obtained should be as 'physiological' as possible. In most cases, effective concentrations achieved in vitro cannot be compared with therapeutic concentrations, since drug binding to proteins cannot be accurately reproduced. This is an important issue for NSAIDs, where $\geq 95\%$ binding to plasma proteins can be observed. However, the human whole blood assay may allow an appropriate representation of in vivo

Figure 2 Selectivity ratios obtained for several NSAIDs using a whole cell assay (dark grey bars)[16,17] or a human whole blood assay (black bars)[18–22,31]. The relatively low values obtained in the whole blood assay for L-745,337 and SC-58125 (hatched bars) are only estimates. Exact ratios cannot be determined because IC$_{50}$ values for COX-1 inhibition were not obtained due to solubility problems at high concentrations.

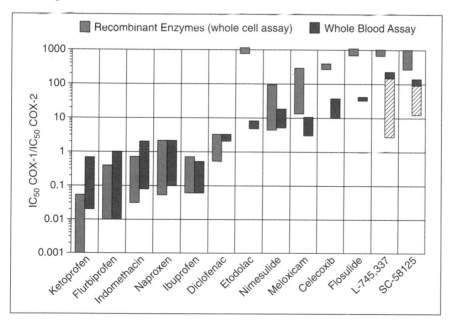

interactions. The concentration–response curves for the inhibition of COX-1 and COX-2 by meloxicam in a human whole blood assay in vitro are shown in Figure 3a. The therapeutic concentrations of meloxicam at steady state levels are also indicated[31]. Inhibition of COX-1 and COX-2 is dependent on the dose; 7.5 mg/day meloxicam is COX-1 sparing and 15 mg/day inhibits COX-1 activity by ~30%. A similar simulation has been constructed for a standard NSAID, indomethacin[32] (Figure 3b). It can be seen that at therapeutic concentrations COX-2 is inhibited by ~90%. However, COX-1 is also inhibited by 90%, indicating the non-selective inhibition by indomethacin.

These simulations have been confirmed in two in vivo studies. Stichtenoth et al.[33] demonstrated that platelet aggregation and thromboxane (TXB_2) formation were almost completely inhibited in volunteers receiving 3×25 mg indomethacin while urinary prostaglandin E_2 (PGE_2) (a marker of renal COX-1 activity) was inhibited by ~50%. These parameters were not affected by 7.5 mg meloxicam. Patrono et al. (personal communication) demonstrated that 7.5 mg and 15 mg meloxicam inhibited COX-2 by 51% and 70%, respectively, and COX-1 by 25% and 35%, respectively, in an ex vivo whole blood assay in healthy volunteers. Thus, the simulations obtained with in vitro results from the whole blood assay can be confirmed in vivo.

However, the selectivity ratio of an NSAID is only one consideration. The simulation in Figure 3a also demonstrates that compounds selective for COX-2, but with some COX-1 inhibitory activity, such as meloxicam, etodolac, and nimesulide, will lose their COX-1 sparing effect with increasing doses. In addition, a flat plasma concentration curve is necessary for these compounds to continuously maintain concentrations above the inhibitory concentration for COX-2 but below the inhibitory concentration for COX-1. The drug concentrations in whole blood with 15 mg/day meloxicam and 200 mg twice a day of nimesulide illustrate this point in Figure 4.

In studies using nimesulide in a dose of 100 mg twice a day, either a 50% inhibition[18] or no inhibition[34] of platelet TXB_2 synthesis was obtained in an ex vivo whole blood assay. The steep plasma concentration curves and relatively high peak plasma levels of the compound (Figure 4b) could explain this discrepancy[35,36]. Concentrations that inhibit COX-1 to a significant extent may be temporarily reached at peak plasma levels. Thus, depending on when blood sampling occurs after drug administration, inhibition of COX-1 may or may not be detected. In an interaction study with furosemide, 200 mg twice a day of nimesulide markedly reduced urinary excretion of PGE_2, suggesting that at this dose the COX-1 sparing effect had vanished[37].

NEWLY DEVELOPED ASSAYS

These test systems use human cells that are target cells for either the anti-inflammatory effects or side effects of NSAIDs, such as gastric mucosal cells, chondrocytes or synoviocytes. Standard conditions still need to be established in order to validate these

Figure 3 Comparison of concentration–response curves for COX-1 and COX-2 inhibition by meloxicam (a) with therapeutic concentrations of 7.5 and 15 mg/day[22,32] and indomethacin (b) with therapeutic concentrations of 3×25 mg/day[22,33]. Drug concentrations in whole blood are calculated from plasma concentrations, assuming drug concentrations in red cells are negligible and that haematocrit is 45%[32].

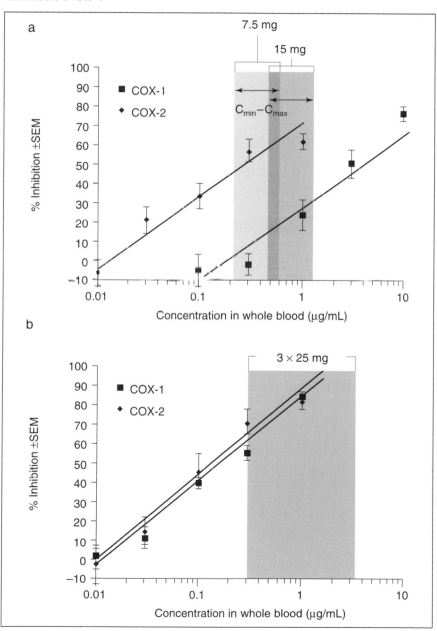

Figure 4 Simulation of drug concentrations in whole blood after repeated administration of meloxicam 15 mg/day (a) and nimesulide 200 mg twice a day (b). IC_{50} values for COX-1 and COX-2 were obtained with the whole blood assay[32,37,38].

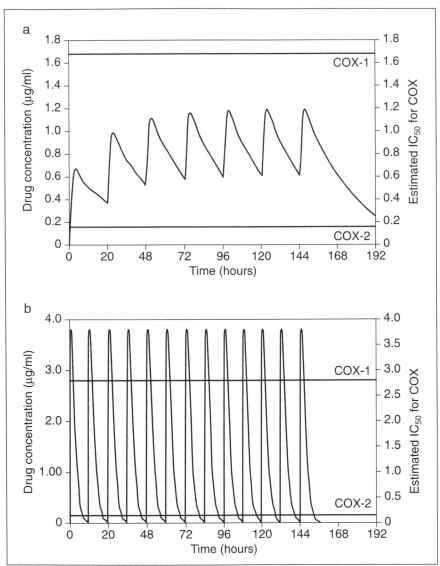

models adequately, and it will also be difficult to mimic drug binding to proteins as closely with these models as in the human whole blood assay. However, a similar trend for ranking of COX-2 selectivity was found for the compounds tested[25–27].

To confirm the in vivo predictive value of these assays, the most relevant markers of COX-1 and COX-2 activity would be the PGE_2 or PGI_2 synthesized by the gastric mucosa and the PGE_2 synthesized by the inflamed synovial tissues, respect-ively[38–41]. In practice, such studies are difficult to perform, since the target tissues are not always easily available. The methods are prone to experimental error, since prostaglandin production can also occur while tissues are being removed at biopsy. Furthermore, prostaglandin concentrations in the gastric fluid or synovial fluid may not precisely reflect the synthetic activity of the gastric mucosa or synovial tissue.

However, promising preliminary results have been obtained by Lapicque et al.[42]. Free (unbound) meloxicam concentrations were measured in the synovial fluid of patients with rheumatoid conditions after administration of a single dose of 15 mg of meloxicam. Figure 5 illustrates the pharmacokinetics of meloxicam in the synovial fluid. In addition, the IC_{50} for COX-2 inhibition measured in vitro with IL-1-stimulated synoviocytes (0.7 ng/ml) is also illustrated[26]. Thus, new approaches to determining the in vivo relevance of COX-2 inhibition by an NSAID in vitro are under way. However, more compounds need to be tested using these methods before the in vivo relevance can be confirmed.

CONCLUSION

Despite the numerous in vitro assays available and the variable results produced by these systems, NSAID selectivity follows a similar trend in the well established models. Results obtained in the human whole blood assay allow NSAIDs to be classified, as: (a) non-selective, (b) COX-2 preferring, and (c) COX-2 selective.

Figure 5 Free meloxicam concentrations in synovial fluid (mean±S.E.M.) in patients receiving a single administration of 15 mg meloxicam[42]. IC_{50} value for COX-2 inhibition determined in IL-1-stimulated synoviocytes[26].

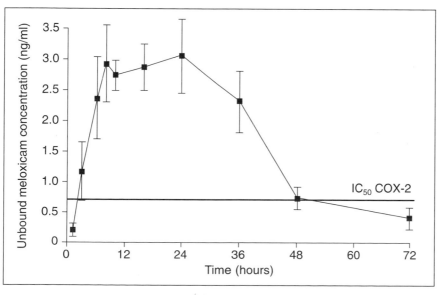

Although in vitro systems are important for measuring inhibitory activity, the clinical relevance of these data needs to be carefully assessed. The level of inhibition of COX-1 and COX-2 in vivo at a particular dose cannot be predicted from in vitro data alone. The pharmacokinetic properties of each compound, including plasma concentrations, whole body distribution and binding to plasma proteins, have to be taken into account. In addition, the definitive test of the therapeutic relevance of COX-2 selectivity must come from head-to-head comparisons in large-scale clinical trials.

REFERENCES

1. Vane JR. Towards a better aspirin. *Nature.* 1994;367:215–6.
2. Pairet M, Engelhardt G. Distinct isoforms (COX-1 and COX-2) of cyclooxygenase: possible physiological and therapeutic implications. *Fundam Clin Pharmacol.* 1996;10:1–15.
3. Pairet M, van Ryn J. Overview of COX-2 in inflammation: from the biology to the clinic. In: Willoughby D, Tomlinson A, editors. *Inducible Enzymes in the Inflammatory Response.* Basel: Birkhäuser Publishing; 1998: in press.
4. Fu JY, Masferrer JL, Seibert K, Raz A, Needleman P. The induction and suppression of prostaglandin H_2 synthase (cyclooxygenase) in human monocytes. *J Biol Chem.* 1990;265:16737–40.
5. Xie W, Chipman JG, Robertson DL, Erikson RL, Simmons DL. Expression of a mitogen-responsive gene encoding prostaglandin synthase is regulated by mRNA splicing. *Proc Natl Acad Sci USA.* 1991;88:1692–6.
6. Pairet M, van Ryn J, Mauz A, Schierok H, Diederen W, Türck D et al. Differential inhibition of COX-1 and COX-2 by NSAIDs: a summary of results obtained using various test systems. In: Vane J, Botting J, editors. *Selective COX-2 Inhibitors: Pharmacology, Clinical Effects and Therapeutic Potential.* London: Kluwer Academic Publishers and William Harvey Press; 1998:27–46.
7. Mitchell JA, Akarasereenont P, Thiemermann C, Flower RJ, Vane JR. Selectivity of nonsteroidal antiinflammatory drugs as inhibitors of constitutive and inducible cyclooxygenase. *Proc Natl Acad Sci USA.* 1994;90:11693–7.
8. Futaki N, Takahashi S, Yokoyama M, Arai I, Higuchi S, Otomo S. NS-398, a new antiinflammatory agent, selectively inhibits prostaglandin G/H synthase/cyclooxygenase (COX-2) activity in vitro. *Prostaglandins.* 1994;47:55–9.
9. Klein T, Nüsing RM, Pfeilschifter J, Ullrich V. Selective inhibition of cyclooxygenase 2. *Biochem Pharmacol.* 1994;48:1605–10.
10. Engelhardt G, Bögel R, Schnitzler C, Utzmann R. Meloxicam: influence on arachidonic acid metabolism: Part 1. In vitro findings. *Biochem Pharmacol.* 1996;51:21–8.
11. Meade EA, Smith WL, DeWitt DL. Differential inhibition of prostaglandin endoperoxide synthase (cyclooxygenase) isozymes by aspirin and other non-steroidal anti-inflammatory drugs. *J Biol Chem.* 1993;268:6610–4.
12. Prasit P, Black WC, Chan CC, Ford-Hutchinson AW, Gauthier JY, Gordon R et al. L-745,337: a selective cyclooxygenase-2 inhibitor. *Med Chem Res.* 1995;5:364–74.
13. Copeland RA, Williams JM, Giannaras J, Nurnberg S, Covington M, Pinto D et al. Mechanism of selective inhibition of the inducible form of prostaglandin G/H synthase. *Proc Natl Acad Sci USA.* 1994;91:11202–6.
14. O'Neill GP, Mancini JA, Kargman S, Yergey J, Kwan MY, Falgueyret JP et al. Overexpression of human prostaglandin G/H synthase-1 and -2 by recombinant vaccinia

virus: inhibition by nonsteroidal anti-inflammatory drugs and biosynthesis of 15-hydroxy-eicosatetraenoic acid. *Mol Pharmacol*. 1994;45:245–54.

15. Glaser K, Sung ML, O'Neill K, Belfast M, Hartman D, Carlson R et al. Etodolac selectively inhibits human prostaglandin G/H synthase 2 (PGHS-2) versus human PGHS-1. *Eur J Pharmacol*. 1995;281:107–11.

16. Churchill L, Graham AG, Shih CK, Pauletti D, Farina PR, Grob PM. Selective inhibition of human cyclo-oxygenase-2 by meloxicam. *Inflammopharmacology*. 1996;4:125–35.

17. Riendeau D, Percival MD, Boyce S, Brideau C, Charleson S, Cromlish W et al. Biochemical and pharmacological profile of a tetrasubstituted furanone as a highly selective COX-2 inhibitor. *Br J Pharmacol*. 1997;121:105–17.

18. Patrignani P, Panara MR, Santini G, Sciulli MG, Padovano R, Cipollone F et al. Differential inhibition of cyclooxygenase activity of prostaglandin endoperoxide synthase isozymes in vitro and ex vivo in man. *Prostaglandins Leukot Essent Fatty Acids*. 1996;55(suppl 1):P115.

19. Young JM, Panah S, Satchawatcharaphong C, Cheung PS. Human whole blood assays for inhibition of prostaglandin G/H synthases-1 and -2 using A23187 and lipopolysaccharide stimulation of thromboxane B_2 production. *Inflamm Res*. 1996;45:246–53.

20. Brideau C, Kargman S, Liu S, Dallob AL, Ehrich EW, Rodger IW et al. A human whole blood assay for clinical evaluation of biochemical efficacy of cyclooxygenase inhibitors. *Inflamm Res*. 1996;45:68–74.

21. Prasit P. New highly selective COX-2 inhibitors. William Harvey Research Conference: Selective COX-2 Inhibitors. Phuket, Sept 18–19, 1997.

22. Pairet M, van Ryn J, Schierok H, Mauz A, Trummlitz G, Engelhardt G. Differential inhibition of cyclooxygenases-1 and -2 by meloxicam and its 4' isomer. *Inflamm Res*. 1998; in press.

23. Warner T. Differential inhibition of COX-1/COX-2 by NSAIDs in human systems. William Harvey Research Conference: Selective COX-2 Inhibitors. Phuket, Sept 18–19, 1997.

24. Tavares IA, Bishai PM, Bennett A. Activity of nimesulide on constitutive and inducible cyclooxygenases. *Arzneimittelforschung*. 1995;45:1093–5.

25. Blanco F, Guitian R, Moreno J, Hernandez A, Freire M, Atanes A et al. NSAID effects on COX-1 and COX-2 activity in human articular chondrocytes. *Arthritis Rheum*. 1997;40(suppl 9):Abstract 347.

26. Vergne P, Bertin P, Liagre B, Bonnet C, Pairet M, Rigaud M et al. Differential inhibition of COX-1 and COX-2 by nonsteroidal antiinflammatory drugs in cultured synovial cells. *Arthritis Rheum*. 1997;40(suppl 9):Abstract 375.

27. Kawai S, Nishida S, Kato M, Furumaya Y, Okamoto R, Koshino T et al. Comparison of cyclooxygenase-1 and -2 inhibitory activities of various nonsteroidal anti-inflammatory drugs using human synovial cells and platelets. 19th ILAR Congress of Rheumatology, Singapore, June 8–13, 1997. Abstract p 156.

28. Hayllar J, Bjarnason I. NSAIDs, COX-2 inhibitors, and the gut. *Lancet*. 1995;346:521–2.

29. Rabasseda X. Nimesulide: a selective cyclooxygenase 2 inhibitor antiinflammatory drug. *Drugs Today*. 1996;32(suppl D):1–23.

30. Cipollone F, Ganci A, Panara MR, Greco A, Cuccurullo F, Patrono C et al. Effects of nabumetone on prostanoid biosynthesis in humans. *Clin Pharmacol Ther*. 1995;58:335–41.

31. Türck D, Busch U, Heinzel G, Narjes HH. Clinical pharmacokinetics of meloxicam. *Arzneimittelforschung*. 1997;47:253–8.

32. McElnay JC, Passmore AP, Crawford VLS, McConnel JG, Taylor IC, Walker FS. Steady state pharmacokinetic profile of indomethacin in elderly patients and young volunteers. *Eur J Clin Pharmacol*. 1992;43:77–80.

33. Stichtenoth DO, Wagner B, Frölich JC. Effects of meloxicam and indomethacin on cyclooxygenase pathways in healthy volunteers. *J Invest Med*. 1997;45:44–9.

34. Cullen L, Kelly L, Coyle D, Forde R, Fitzgerald D. Selective suppression of COX-2 during chronic administration of nimesulide in man. William Harvey Research Conference: Selective COX-2 Inhibitors; Pharmacology, Clinical Effects and Therapeutic Potential, Cannes, March 20–21, 1997, Abstract P3.

35. Theiss U, Timmer W, Wieckhorst G, Macciocchi A, Wetzelsberger N. Investigation into possible drug–drug interaction between warfarin and nimesulide in healthy volunteers. *Methods Find Exp Clin Pharmacol*. 1993;15:629–35.

36. Davis R, Bodgen RN. Nimesulide. An update of its pharmacodynamic and pharmacokinetic properties, and therapeutic efficacy. *Drugs*. 1994;48:431–54.

37. Steinhäuslin F, Munajo A, Buclin T, Macciochi A, Biollaz J. Renal effects of nimesulide in furosemide-treated subjects. Drugs. 1993;46(suppl 1):257–62.

38. Russell RI. Endoscopic evaluation of etodolac and naproxen and their relative effects on gastric and duodenal prostaglandins. *Rheumatol Int*. 1990;10:17–21.

39. Day RO, Francis H, Vial J, Geisslinger G, Williams KM. Naproxen concentrations in plasma and synovial fluid and effects on prostanoid concentrations. *J Rheumatol*. 1995;22:2295–303.

40. Hudson N, Balsitis M, Filipowicz F, Hawkey C. Effect of Helicobacter pylori colonisation on gastric mucosal eicosanoid synthesis in patients taking non-steroidal anti-inflammatory drugs. *Gut*. 1993;34:748–51.

41. Bertin P, Lapicque F, Payan E, Rigaud M, Bailleul F, Jaeger S et al. Sodium naproxen: concentration and effect on inflammatory response mediators in human rheumatoid synovial fluid. *Clin Pharmacol*. 1994;46:3–7.

42. Lapicque F, Gillet P, Guillaume C, Vignon E, Thomas P, Velicitat P et al. Diffusion of meloxicam into synovial fluid after a single oral dose. Effect of inflammation and gender. *J Pharmacol Exp Ther*. 1998;submitted.

3

Differential target tissue presentation and cyclooxygenase-2 and -1 inhibition by non-steroidal anti-inflammatory drugs

H. FENNER

Non-steroidal anti-inflammatory drugs (NSAIDs) are widely used for the treatment of rheumatoid arthritis and osteoarthritis in patients who require long-term management of pain and inflammatory synovitis. The use of these drugs has, however, traditionally been associated with gastrointestinal (GI) side effects, presenting a significant problem for this group of patients. Anecdotal evidence has suggested that the NSAIDs differ in their degree of gut toxicity. However, only recent pharmaco-epidemiological studies have given a realistic indication of the risk of serious GI complications associated with individual agents[1-4].

It was originally thought that inhibition of cyclooxygenase (COX) was responsible for both the therapeutic and toxic effects of NSAIDs[5]. However, the recent discovery of two distinct isoforms of this enzyme[6] has enabled the mechanism of action of NSAIDs to be further elucidated.

The tissue distribution of COX activity has been found to be different for the two isoforms. COX-1 is constitutively expressed in most cells/tissues, including platelets, gastric mucosa and kidney[7]. COX-1-derived prostanoids regulate platelet aggregation and the integrity and function of the gut mucosa and kidney respectively[8]. Thus, one would predict that inhibition of COX-1 would result in detrimental effects on these cells and tissues. In contrast, COX-2, which is expressed in various cell types, such as monocytes, fibroblasts and synovial cells, is induced in response to inflammatory stimuli[9]. Agents which inhibit COX-2 should, therefore, have anti-inflammatory effects.

The traditionally-used NSAIDs inhibit both COX isoforms simultaneously, in vitro and ex vivo, but have been found to inhibit the two isoforms to different extents, suggesting differences in their beneficial anti-inflammatory and detrimental effects. One approach to quantifying the effects at the cellular or tissue level is based on: (1) the inherent potency of the agent towards the target enzyme located in the cell/tissue of interest (pharmacodynamic profile), and (2) the drug concentration/time course, which determines drug exposure of target cells/tissues (pharmacokinetic profile).

The pharmacokinetic and pharmacodynamic profiles of NSAIDs should be characterized not only in the synovial ('anti-inflammatory effect') and GI ('toxicity') compartments but also at the level of tissue exposure, i.e. synovial tissue and GI mucosa. This would enable the concentration/time course of the drug presentation to cells/tissues expressing either COX isoform to be determined. Unfortunately, as such data are not presently available for most NSAIDs, surrogate systems have to be applied.

This chapter discusses the methodology for determining pharmacodynamic and pharmacokinetic profiles of NSAIDs. The rationale for integrating these profiles for NSAIDs will be explained with the use of specific NSAIDs as examples.

PHARMACODYNAMIC DRUG PROFILES

The pharmacodynamic drug profile denotes the relative selectivity of an NSAID for COX-1 and COX-2. The selectivity of NSAIDs for the COX isoforms has been studied in a variety of experimental models, including purified enzyme systems, cell systems incorporating human recombinant enzymes, non-human cells, such as guinea pig macrophages, and human whole blood assays[10-13]. Classical NSAIDs have been shown to inhibit both isoforms non-selectively or to be preferentially COX-1 selective.

The pharmacodynamic drug profiles of NSAIDs can be determined in human whole blood by measuring their in vitro inhibitory effect on the activity of COX-1 in platelets and COX-2 in monocytes[9,10,13-15]. Inhibition of the formation of thromboxane A_2 by NSAIDs is used as a measure of COX-1 inhibitory activity, whereas the inhibition of COX-2 is determined by measuring the effects of NSAIDs on prostaglandin E_2 formation in lipopolysaccharide-stimulated monocytes. From these data, dose–response curves can be generated allowing the IC_{50} (NSAID concentration producing 50% inhibition) to be calculated for COX-1 and COX-2[16-25].

Human whole blood assays more accurately reflect the physiological and therapeutic situation than most other experimental systems used for testing differential COX inhibition. The whole blood model is a valid predictor of both drug presentation and effects at the level of COX expression in intracellular lipid membranes as: (1) only the free fraction of the drug is distributed into the target cell (platelet or monocyte), and (2) differences between drugs with respect to physicochemical features, transmembrane transfer and the kinetics of the drug–COX enzyme interaction are reflected by the target tissue concentration.

PHARMACOKINETIC DRUG PROFILES

The pharmacokinetic profile of an NSAID is determined by measuring the concentration/time course of the drug in the compartments which express the two COX isoforms. As there is a marked expression of COX-2 in inflamed human synovium[26], this suggests that distribution of the drug into the synovial compartment could be an important predictor of efficacy. Similarly, distribution of the drug into sites of COX-1 expression, such as platelets, may predict GI and kidney toxicity.

Data on the pharmacokinetic profiles of NSAIDs are available from a number of previously published and other studies[16–25]. The drug concentration/time profiles in the synovial and systemic compartments are used as surrogates for respective drug concentrations in synovial tissue and GI mucosa. They logically correlate with drug activity in the adjacent cellular microenvironment and reflect the tissue distribution and target enzyme kinetics (Figure 1).

The pharmacokinetic profile, at the synovial cell level, determines the time course of intracellular drug presentation to COX-2 located in the lipid layers. In this rationale, it is assumed that a direct and constant relationship exists between the concentration of a drug at therapeutic dose levels in the synovial fluid and in the adjacent tissues. Thus, the synovial fluid/plasma concentration/time course is a measure of the relative NSAID concentration in the two compartments. This can be expressed by the ratio of the area under the curve (AUC) synovial fluid/AUC plasma (whole blood).

Figure I NSAID presentation to target synovial and systemic compartments

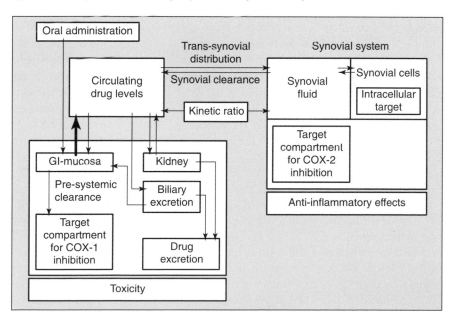

The concentration/time course for both the synovial and systemic compartments in relation to onset, magnitude and duration of COX inhibitory effects is reflected by C_{max}, C_{min} and C_{mean} in synovial fluid and whole blood. A high synovial fluid/plasma ratio reflects the potential for synovial COX-2 inhibition relative to systemic COX-1, whereas a low ratio means higher drug concentrations in the tissues where COX-1 is expressed.

INTEGRATION OF PHARMACOKINETIC AND PHARMACODYNAMIC PROFILES OF NSAIDS

Ideally, NSAID profiles should be assessed in patients by simultaneous measurement of COX activity in biopsy specimens taken from the GI mucosa and from synovial tissue. However, this is difficult to perform for practical and ethical reasons, and surrogate measures are used which describe the drug profile as closely as possible to the ideal. These drug profiles define the NSAID concentration/time course in the synovial compartment and the corresponding inhibitory effect on COX-2-expressing synovial cells. This is relative to the concentration/time course in the systemic compartment and the inhibitory effect on COX-1-expressing cells.

Integration of pharmacokinetic data into dose–response curves provides information on differential COX-2/COX-1 inhibitory activity at therapeutic drug concentrations. Such integration can be achieved by two different approaches: (1) 'reading-out' in vitro dose–response curves, and (2) pharmacodynamic modelling using the E_{max} model[27].

'Reading-out' In Vitro Dose–Response Curves
A 'read-out' from dose–response curves for meloxicam and naproxen which were generated from an in vitro whole blood assay enabled the COX-2 inhibitory activity in the synovial compartment to be calculated in this laboratory. Also it allowed the measurement of COX-1 inhibitory activity in whole blood at therapeutic drug concentrations. Inhibition of COX-2 ranged from 72 to 85% for both naproxen (500 mg) and meloxicam (15 mg), whereas COX-1 inhibition was much less with meloxicam (12–36%) than naproxen (86–94%).

Pharmacodynamic Modelling
Integration of pharmacokinetic data into the pharmacodynamic profile using the E_{max} model has enabled the COX-2 inhibitory activity, relative to COX-1 inhibition, to be calculated for all NSAIDs in the whole blood assay (Figure 2). This has allowed the intrinsic potency of particular NSAIDs to inhibit synovial COX-2 relative to systemic COX-1 to be calculated at different time points.

The data in Tables 1 and 2 show that NSAIDs have different inhibitory activities for COX-1 at different time points, whereas no major differences are observed in their COX-2 inhibitory activities. An exception is nabumetone, as at the recommended daily dose (1 g) this agent inhibits both COX isoforms to the

Figure 2 *Pharmacodynamic modelling (LPS=bacterial lipopolysaccharide)*

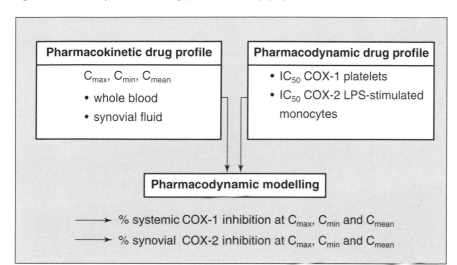

same extent (30–40%). Nabumetone has also been studied using the ex vivo model, which uses blood samples from volunteers who have taken NSAIDs in therapeutic doses over a number of days[28]. This study demonstrated that nabumetone inhibited both isoforms non-selectively[28].

SUMMARY

The recent discovery of two isoforms of the COX enzyme has led to the COX concept being put forward as one approach to improving the outcome of patients taking NSAIDs. The concept predicts that the inhibition of COX-1 by NSAIDs may result in unwanted GI and renal side effects, whereas inhibition of COX-2 may underlie the beneficial, anti-inflammatory effects of these drugs. Meloxicam is an NSAID which preferentially inhibits COX-2 relative to COX-1. Meloxicam has been shown in double-blind trials to be as effective as classical NSAIDs in the treatment of osteoarthritis and rheumatoid arthritis[29]. Furthermore, in a global analysis of clinical trials and two large-scale 28-day studies, meloxicam was shown to have an improved GI toxicity profile in comparison with classical NSAIDs[30–32].

As the two COX isoforms are expressed in separate physiological/pathophysiological compartments, it is possible to integrate data from concentration/time courses of NSAIDs in the synovial/systemic compartments (pharmacokinetic profile) and the selectivity for COX-2/COX-1 (pharmacodynamic profile). This enables the concentration/time course of the drug presentation to the cells/tissues expressing the two COX isoforms to be determined. In the treatment of arthritic disease the efficacy of an NSAID would be expected to result from the inhibition of synovial COX-2, whereas one would predict that the toxicity would be

Table 1 Whole blood concentration and COX-1 inhibition by NSAIDs at different drug concentrations

NSAID	IC_{50} COX-1 (µg/ml)	NSAID dose	C_{max} (µg/ml) [h]	COX-1 inhibition (%)	C_{min} (µg/ml) [h]	COX-1 inhibition (%)	C_{mean} (µg/ml) [h]	COX-1 inhibition (%)	Reference
Diclofenac	0.045 (reference 14)	50 mg tid	0.44 [3]	91	0.034 [8]	43			17
		100 mg SR md					0.06–0.12 [4–8]	57–73	18
Indomethacin	0.06	50 mg md	1.6 [1]	96	0.19 [9]	76	0.22–0.33 [3–7]	78–84	16
(S) Ketoprofen	0.03	200 mg SR md	0.8 [6–8]	96	0.17 [24]	85	0.5	94	19
Meloxicam	1.7	15 mg md	1.1 [5]	39	0.4 [24]	19	0.8 [5–14]	32	24
Nabumetone	60	1 g/day md	72	55	23 [24]	28	41	41	21
Naproxen	3.6	500 mg bid md	49 [2]	93	23 [12]	87	35	91	22
Piroxicam	0.95	20 mg md	4.4 [3]	82	2.5 [24]	73	3.5	79	20

bid=twice daily; tid=three times daily; md=multiple dose; SR=slow release

Table 2 Synovial fluid concentration and COX-2 inhibition by NSAIDs at different drug concentrations

NSAID	IC_{50} COX-2 (μg/ml)	NSAID dose	C_{max} (mg/ml) [h]	COX-2 inhibition (%)	C_{min} (μg/ml) [h]	COX-2 inhibition (%)	C_{mean} (μg/ml) [h]	COX-2 inhibition (%)	Reference
Diclofenac	0.016 (reference 14)	50 mg tid	0.16 [3]	91	0.09 [8]	85			17
		100 mg SR md	0.10 [4]	86	0.035 [16–21]	69	0.07	81	18
Indomethacin	0.05	50 mg md	0.38 [2]	88	0.22 [9]	82	0.3	86	16
(S) Ketoprofen	0.046	200 mg SR md	0.6 [7]	93	0.4 [24]	90	0.5	92	19
Meloxicam	0.15	15 mg md	0.55 [5]	88	0.33 [24]	81	0.46	86	23, 25
Nabumetone	40	1 g/day md					19	32	21
Naproxen	6.4	500 mg bid md	26 [5]	80	17 [12]	73	21.5	77	22
Piroxicam	0.3	20 mg md	0.3 [6]	91	1.7 [24]	85	2.4	89	20

bid=twice daily; tid=three times daily; md=multiple dose; SR=slow release attributed to inhibition of systemic COX-1 activity. Such application of drug concentration/time profiles of individual agents may help to enable the onset, magnitude and duration of their characteristic COX-inhibitory effects to be predicted.

REFERENCES

1. Fries JF, Williams CA, Bloch DA. The relative toxicity of nonsteroidal antiinflammatory drugs. *Arthritis Rheum*. 1991;34:1353–60.
2. Henry D, Dobson A, Turner C. Variability in the risk of major gastrointestinal complications from nonaspirin nonsteroidal anti-inflammatory drugs. *Gastroenterology*. 1993; 105:1078–88.
3. García Rodríguez LA, Jick H. Risk of upper gastrointestinal bleeding and perforation associated with individual non-steroidal anti-inflammatory drugs. *Lancet*. 1994;343:769–72.
4. Langman MJS. Anti-inflammatory drugs and the gut: ulcerative damage and protection from cancer. *Proceedings of Symposium: New Insights into Antiinflammatory Therapy and its Benefits*. Cannes, October, 1994.
5. Vane JR. Inhibition of prostaglandin synthesis as a mechanism of action for the aspirin-like drugs. *Nat New Biol*. 1971;231:232–5.
6. Masferrer JL, Zweifel BS, Seibert K, Needleman P. Selective regulation of cellular cyclooxygenase by dexamethasone and endotoxin in mice. *J Clin Invest*. 1990;86:1375–9.
7. Patrignani P, Panara MR, Greco A, Fusco O, Natoli C, Iacobelli S et al. Biochemical and pharmacological characterization of the cyclooxygenase activity of human blood prostaglandin endoperoxide synthases. *J Pharmacol Exp Ther*. 1994;271:1705–12.
8. Vane J. Towards a better aspirin. *Nature*. 1994;367:215–6.
9. Pairet M, Engelhardt G. Differential inhibition of COX-1 and COX-2 in vitro and pharmacokinetic profile in vivo of NSAIDs. In: Vane J, Botting J, Botting R, editors. *Improved Non-Steroid Anti-Inflammatory Drugs – COX-2 Enzyme Inhibitors*. London: Kluwer Academic Publishing and William Harvey Press; 1996:103–19.
10. Glaser KB. Cyclooxygenase selectivity and NSAIDs: Cyclooxygenase-2 selectivity of etodolac (Lodine). *Inflammopharmacology*. 1995;3:335–45.
11. Churchill L, Graham AG, Shih C-K, Pauletti D, Farina PR, Grob PM. Selective inhibition of human cyclo-oxygenase-2 by meloxicam. *Inflammopharmacology*. 1996;4:125–35.
12. Engelhardt G, Bögel R, Schnitzer Chr, Utzmann R. Meloxicam: influence on arachidonic acid metabolism. Part 1. In vitro findings. *Biochem Pharmacol*. 1996;51:21–8.
13. Patrignani P, Panara MR, Santini G, Sciulli MG, Padovano R, Cipollone F et al. Differential inhibition of the cyclooxygenase activity of prostaglandin endoperoxide synthase isozymes in vitro and ex vivo in man. *Prostaglandins Leukot Essent Fatty Acids*. 1996;55(suppl 1):98 Abstr P115.
14. Brideau C, Kargman S, Liu S, Dallob AL, Ehrich EW, Rodger IW et al. A human whole blood assay for clinical evaluation of biochemical efficacy of cyclooxygenase inhibitors. *Inflamm Res*. 1996;45:68–74.
15. Young JM, Panah S, Satchawatcharaphong C, Cheung PS. Human whole blood assays for inhibition of prostaglandin G/H synthases-1 and -2 using A23187 and lipopolysaccharide stimulation of thromboxane B_2 production. *Inflamm Res*. 1996;45:246–53.
16. Emori WE, Champion GD, Bluestone R, Paulus HE. Simultaneous pharmacokinetics of indomethacin in serum and synovial fluid. *Ann Rheum Dis*. 1973;32:433–5.
17. Fowler PD, Shadforth MF, Crook PR, John VA. Plasma and synovial fluid concentrations of diclofenac sodium and its major hydroxylated metabolites during long-term treatment of rheumatoid arthritis. *Eur J Clin Pharmacol*. 1983;25:389–94.

18. Fowler PD, Dawes PT, John VA, Shotton PA. Plasma and synovial fluid concentrations of diclofenac sodium and its hydroxylated metabolites during once-daily administration of a 100 mg slow-release formulation. *Eur J Clin Pharmacol.* 1986;31:469–72.

19. McCrea JD, Telford AM, Kaye CM, Boyd MW. A comparison of plasma and synovial fluid profiles of standard and controlled-release formulations of ketoprofen in patients with rheumatoid arthritis. *Curr Med Res Opin.* 1986;10:73–81.

20. Kurowski M, Dunky A. Transsynovial kinetics of piroxicam in patients with rheumatoid arthritis. *Eur J Clin Pharmacol.* 1988;34:401–6.

21. Miehlke RK, Schneider S, Sorgel F, Muth P, Henschke F, Giersch KH et al. Penetration of the active metabolite of nabumetone into synovial fluid and adherent tissue of patients undergoing knee joint surgery. *Drugs.* 1990;40(suppl 5):57–61.

22. Day RO, Francis H, Vial J, Geisslinger G, Williams KM. Naproxen concentrations in plasma and synovial fluid and effects on prostanoid concentrations. *J Rheumatol.* 1995;22:2295–303.

23. Degner F, Heinzel G, Busch U. Transsynovial kinetics of meloxicam. *Scand J Rheumatol.* 1994;(suppl 98):Abstr 121.

24. Türck D, Busch U, Heinzel G, Narjes H. Clinical pharmacokinetics of meloxicam. *Arzneimittelforschung.* 1997;47:253–8.

25. Lapicque F, Gillet P, Vignon, E, Thomas P, Velicitat P, Tuerk D et al. Effect of inflammation on meloxicam diffusion into synovial fluid (SF) after a single oral dose. *Clin. Pharmacol. Ther.* 1998;63:167,Abstr PiI–122.

26. Crofford LJ. COX-1 and COX-2 tissue expression: implications and predictions. *J Rheumatol.* 1997;24(suppl 49):15–19.

27. Schwinghammer TL, Kroboth PD. Basic concepts in pharmaco-dynamic modeling. *J Clin Pharmacol.* 1988;28:388–94.

28. Cipollone F, Ganci A, Panara MR, Greco A, Cuccurullo F, Patrono C et al. Effects of nabumetone on prostanoid biosynthesis in humans. *Clin Pharmacol Ther.* 1995;58:335–41.

29. Barner A. Review of clinical trials and benefit/risk ratio of meloxicam. *Scand J Rheumatol.* 1996;25(suppl 102):29–37.

30. Distel M, Mueller C, Bluhmki E, Fries J. Safety of meloxicam: a global analysis of clinical trials. *Br J Rheumatol.* 1996;35(suppl 1):68–77.

31. Dequeker J, Hawkey C, Kahan A, Alegre C, Baumelou E, Bégaud B et al. Improvement in gastrointestinal tolerability of the selective COX-2 inhibitor, meloxicam, compared with piroxicam: results of the Safety and Efficacy Large-scale Evaluation of COX-inhibiting Therapies (SELECT) trial in osteoarthritis. *Br J Rheumatol.* 1998;37:946–51.

32. Hawkey C, Kahan A, Steinbrück K, Alegre C, Baumelou E, Bégaud B et al. Gastrointestinal tolerability of meloxicam compared to diclofenac in osteoarthritis patients. *Br J Rheumatol.* 1998;37:937–45.

Cyclooxygenase-1 and -2 in synovial tissues of arthritis patients

L. J. CROFFORD

Rheumatoid arthritis (RA) is a systemic inflammatory disease whose dominant clinical feature is symmetrical polyarticular synovitis. Characteristic histopathological changes in RA include infiltration of synovial tissues with mononuclear inflammatory cells, marked proliferation of synovial lining cells and sub-lining fibroblast-like cells, and genesis of new supporting blood vessels. These changes lead to pain and swelling of joints, formation of rheumatoid pannus, and erosion of articular cartilage and juxta-articular bone. Though the aetiology of RA is not known, the pathogenesis involves complex interactions between cells of the immune system and resident cells of the synovia. A number of autocrine and paracrine mediators, including cytokines, growth factors and eicosanoids, are likely to contribute to the proliferative and invasive phenotype of inflamed synovial tissues in RA[1].

PROSTAGLANDINS IN RA

Prostaglandins (PGs) are elevated in the synovial fluids and tissues of patients with RA[2]. PGs mediate the characteristic vasodilatation and erythema seen in acute inflammation. Since vasodilatation increases blood flow in inflamed tissues, PGs contribute to fluid extravasation caused by agents which increase vascular permeability. PGs also sensitize peripheral nociceptors to other mediators that produce inflammatory pain. In addition to mediating classic inflammation in rheumatoid synovial tissues, PGs contribute to phenotypic changes associated with the proliferative and invasive phenotype of pannus. PGE_2 stimulates production of matrix metalloproteinases by synoviocytes that leads to destruction of cartilage and bone[3–5]. In addition, PGE_2 stimulates angiogenesis[6–8], possibly by increasing production of vascular endothelial growth factor in synoviocytes[9]. PGs are multi-functional mediators that have anti-inflammatory as well as pro-inflammatory properties, particularly in leucocytes. By way of example, PGE_2 inhibits lymphocyte proliferation in response to mitogens, lymphocyte-mediated cytotoxicity, cytokine secretion, antibody formation and migration of mono-nuclear cells[10,11]. PGE_2 also inhibits chemotaxis, phagocytosis, degranulation, generation of oxygen-derived free radicals, adherence to endothelium and synthesis of leukotriene B_4 in neutrophils[10,11].

PG Production

PGs are derived primarily from arachidonate hydrolysed from the *sn*-2 position of membrane phospholipids by the action of phospholipase A_2 (PLA_2). Free arachidonate undergoes a cyclooxygenation (COX) reaction to form PGG_2, then a peroxidation reaction in which PGG_2 undergoes reduction to form the endoperoxide, PGH_2. Both enzymatic functions are performed by COX. COX-1 is the constitutively expressed form of the enzyme, while COX-2 is rapidly and markedly increased in vivo and in vitro in response to many extracellular stimuli[12]. PGH_2 is rapidly metabolized by one of the PG synthases. PGE_2 is the predominant PG in synovial fluids and tissues, and is formed by a non-oxidative isomerization by PGE synthase[13].

The COX Enzymes

There are two isoforms of COX, COX-1 and COX-2. It has been proposed that COX-1 and COX-2 subserve different physiological functions largely because of the striking differences in their tissue expression and regulation. COX-1 displays the characteristics of a 'housekeeping' gene, and the promoter displays little significant inducible transcription[12]. Accordingly, COX-1 is constitutively expressed in almost all tissues, including synovial tissues. In sharp contrast, COX-2 is an 'immediate-early' gene that is rapidly inducible and tightly regulated (Table 1). Under basal conditions, COX-2 expression is highly restricted, with the highest levels of expression in the brain and kidney. COX-2 expression is dramatically increased during inflammation and dysregulated proliferation.

Table 1 Regulation of COX-2 expression

Increased COX-2
• Pro-inflammatory cytokines: IL-1, TNF-α, LPS
• Mitogens: serum, phorbol esters
• Growth factors: PDGF, TGF-β, EGF, FGF, GM-CSF
• Cell–cell interactions: CD40–CD40 ligand

Decreased COX-2
• Glucocorticoids
• Anti-inflammatory cytokines: IL-4, IL-13, IL-10

IL=interleukin; TNF=tumour necrosis factor; LPS=lipopolysaccharide; PDGF=platelet-derived growth factor; TGF=transforming growth factor; EGF=epidermal growth factor; FGF=fibroblast growth factor; GM-CSF=granulocyte–macrophage colony stimulating factor

Pro-inflammatory cytokines, such as tumour necrosis factor (TNF)-α and interleukin (IL)-1, increase COX-2 expression in virtually all cytokine-sensitive cell types evaluated to date, including synoviocytes, vascular endothelial cells, chondrocytes, osteoblasts, and monocyte/macrophages[14–21]. The promoter of the human COX-2 gene contains a number of potential binding sites for transcription factors commonly seen in the promoter regions of highly regulated genes, particularly those that are upregulated during inflammation (Figure 1)[22]. Several of these transcription factors are known to be stimulated by IL-1 and/or TNF-α, including NF-κB, CCAAT/enhancer binding protein (c/EBP, also known as nuclear factor for IL-6 or NF-IL6), and the cyclic AMP responsive element binding protein (CREBP). All of these transcription factors have been shown to be involved in stimulated COX-2 transcription in certain cell types. In synoviocytes, IL-1β stimulates NF-κB translocation to the nucleus and binding to the COX-2 promoter stimulates transcription[23].

Two γ-interferon-activated sequence motifs (GAS) are present in the human COX-2 promoter (Figure 1)[24]. Accumulating data suggest that COX-2 expression may be modulated by cytokine networks involving signal transducers and activators of transcription[24].

Mitogenic stimuli and growth factors are also important regulators of COX-2. Platelet-derived growth factor (PDGF) stimulates COX-2 expression in mouse 3T3 cells via Ras-dependent signal transduction pathways[25]. Though similar results have not yet been reported in synoviocytes, PDGF is the principal synoviocyte growth factor.

It has recently been demonstrated that interaction of CD40 and CD40 ligand stimulates COX-2 expression in human lung fibroblasts[26]. Expression of CD40

Figure 1 Transcription factor binding sites in the COX-2 and COX-1 promoters. The COX-2 promoter contains binding sites for multiple transcription factors associated with rapidly inducible tightly regulated genes, particularly those up-regulated during inflammation. The COX-1 promoter has the characteristics of a 'housekeeping' gene, lacking a TATA-box and having few binding sites for inducible transcription factors.

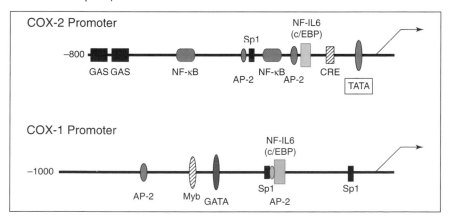

on rheumatoid synoviocytes has been demonstrated, making this mechanism for regulation of COX-2 in RA plausible[27].

COX-2 is downregulated by glucocorticoids (GC) in all tissues examined to date in vivo and in vitro[14,17,21,28–31]. GC inhibit COX-2 expression by transcriptional mechanisms through interactions with the GC receptor[32], and post-transcriptional mechanisms may also be operative.

COX EXPRESSION AND REGULATION IN ANIMAL MODELS OF ARTHRITIS

We evaluated expression of COX in joint tissues of LEW rats over time after intraperitoneal injection of streptococcal cell walls or intradermal injection of Freund's complete adjuvant[31]. These animal studies were performed prior to the characterization of the COX-2 isoform, and the antisera used recognize *both* COX-1 and -2. Nevertheless, there was little immunostaining for COX in untreated animals, and markedly increased expression of immunoreactive COX that preceded the development of clinical arthritis. COX immunostaining was detected in multiple cell types within the joints and surrounding tissues.

Anderson and co-workers extended our work by performing specific COX isoform analysis of rats with adjuvant-induced arthritis[28]. They confirmed that COX-2, but not COX-1, mRNA increased concomitantly with, or just prior to, the onset of detectable paw swelling. Increased expression of COX-2 mRNA was followed by increased COX-2 protein expression and tissue PGE_2 levels. Furthermore, treatment of arthritic animals with the specific COX-2 inhibitor, SC-58125 (Searle, St Louis, MO, USA) suppressed paw swelling by 80–85%. This level of suppression was equivalent to indomethacin, which inhibits both COX isoforms, while dexamethasone (DEX) inhibited paw oedema by 95–100%[28].

COX EXPRESSION IN SYNOVIA OF PATIENTS WITH ARTHRITIS

Using a polyclonal antibody that recognized *both* COX-1 and -2, we examined COX expression by immunohistochemical staining of synovial tissues from patients with RA, osteoarthritis (OA), and non-arthritic patients with traumatic injury[31]. Synovial tissues from patients with RA exhibited intense staining of the synovial lining layer, sub-synovial synoviocytes, vascular endothelial cells, and mononuclear inflammatory cells. The extent and intensity of COX immunostaining correlated with the degree of mononuclear cell infiltration that provided a measure of the synovial inflammation. COX immunostaining was less intense in patients with OA, and there was little immunoreactive COX detected in non-arthritic synovial tissues.

An antibody specific for the unique carboxy-terminal peptide of human COX-2 was generated and used for immunostaining of rheumatoid synovial tissues[14]. COX-2 immunostaining was prominent in vascular endothelial cells, infiltrating mononuclear inflammatory cells, and sub-lining synoviocytes. COX-1 and -2 transcripts were detected in synovial tissues of RA patients by reverse transcriptase polymerase chain reaction (RT-PCR) analysis. More recently, Siegle et al. demonstrated immunostaining for both COX-1 and -2 in patients with RA, seronegative inflammatory arthritis and OA[33]. Expression of COX-1 was most clearly demonstrated in the synovial lining layer, and was not linked to inflammatory arthritis. COX-2 immunostaining was increased in the blood vessel endothelial cells, lining layer, and sublining layer in patients with inflammatory arthritis compared with OA. They also demonstrated elevated COX-2 mRNA expression in RA compared with OA[33]. The finding of ongoing COX-2 mRNA expression in patients with long-standing disease undergoing joint replacement surgery indicates ongoing stimuli for synthesis of COX-2 or failure to appropriately suppress transcription.

COX EXPRESSION AND REGULATION IN SYNOVIAL TISSUES IN VITRO

In vitro analysis of cultured human synovial tissues has contributed to the understanding of factors that regulate expression of COX. We evaluated the expression and regulation of COX-1 and -2 protein in fresh explants of rheumatoid synovia[14]. These synovial explant tissues contain macrophage-like and fibroblast-like synovial cells, as well as endothelial cells and mononuclear inflammatory cells. COX-1 and -2 were detected by immunoprecipitation of metabolically labelled proteins and by Western blot analysis under basal conditions. Treatment with IL-1β or phorbol ester (PMA) markedly increased expression of COX-2, and pre-treatment with DEX eliminated basal and stimulated COX-2 expression. These treatments had little effect on the level of COX-1 expression.

Since synoviocytes are a major source of PG in rheumatoid synovial tissues, we examined expression and regulation of COX mRNA by Northern blot analysis in primary cultured rheumatoid synoviocytes. A small amount of COX-2 mRNA was seen at baseline. IL-1β, TNF-α, and PMA stimulated COX-2 expression. DEX effectively inhibited stimulated expression. A time course for induction of endogenous COX-2 mRNA by IL-1β demonstrated a rapid rise of endogenous COX-2 message by 30 minutes after stimulation. Northern blot analysis confirmed the RT-PCR result. COX-2 protein increases by 1–2 hours, and high levels of expression are sustained 24 hours after treatment.

Treatment of synoviocytes with the transcription inhibitor, actinomycin-D, completely eliminated basal and stimulated COX-2 mRNA expression; while treatment with cycloheximide, which inhibits translation, markedly increased COX-2 expression. That COX-2 transcription is independent of new protein synthesis is consistent with the notion that COX-2 acts as an immediate-early gene, underlining the importance of COX-2 as an early biological response modifier in these cells.

Although COX-1 mRNA and protein are detectable in RA synovial tissues and cultured synoviocytes, COX-2 is the enzyme responsible for virtually all of the PG production in these tissues in vitro. Synovial explant tissue from a patient with RA was cultured overnight in medium containing acetylsalicylic acid (ASA) or the selective COX-2 inhibitor NS-398[34]. NS-398 was as effective as ASA in blocking basal and IL-1β-stimulated PG production determined by enzyme immunoassay (unpublished observation). In addition, we demonstrated that NS-398 was as effective as ASA in blocking PG production stimulated by either IL-1β or TNF-α in cultured synoviocytes (unpublished observation). It must be remembered, however, that soluble PLA_2 ($sPLA_2$) is present in large amounts in the synovial fluid of RA patients[35]. $sPLA_2$ may provide the substrate for production of PG by COX-1 or -2 in vivo.

TREATMENT IMPLICATIONS OF INCREASED COX-2 EXPRESSION IN ARTHRITIS

Inhibition of PG production has been a mainstay of the treatment of acute inflammation in arthritis patients for centuries. Based on the current understanding of the biology of COX-1 and -2 in inflammatory arthritis, it has been proposed that the beneficial clinical effects of non-steroidal anti-inflammatory drugs are due to inhibition of COX-2, while the most important undesirable side effects of these compounds (gastrointestinal tract (GI) ulceration, inhibition of platelet function) reflect inhibition of COX-1. Based on these expectations, highly selective inhibitors of COX-2 are under development by several pharmaceutical companies. Large-scale clinical trials are necessary to establish that: (1) the selective inhibitors of COX-2 are as effective as non-specific COX inhibitors as anti-inflammatory and analgesic compounds in inflammatory arthritis, (2) the expectation of decreased GI ulceration and bleeding holds true, and (3) no unexpected consequences (i.e. accelerated cartilage loss or osteoporosis, renal effects, effects on reproductive function) of selective COX-2 inhibition are detected. Should these goals be achieved, highly selective inhibition of COX-2 will be a significant advance in the treatment of patients with inflammatory arthritis.

REFERENCES

1. Crofford LJ. Expression and regulation of COX-2 in synovial tissues of arthritis patients. In: Vane J, Botting J, Botting R, editors. *Improved Non-Steroid Anti-Inflammatory Drugs. COX-2 Enzyme Inhibitors.* London: Kluwer Academic Publishers and William Harvey Press; 1996:133–43.
2. Vane JR, Botting RM. Overview – mechanisms of action of anti-inflammatory drugs. In: Vane J, Botting J, Botting R, editors. *Improved Non-Steroid Anti-Inflammatory Drugs.* London: Kluwer Academic Publishers and William Harvey Press; 1996:1–27.
3. Robinson DR, Tashijian AHJ, Levine L. Prostaglandin-stimulated bone resorption by rheumatoid synovia: a possible mechanism for bone destruction in rheumatoid arthritis. *J Clin Invest.* 1975;56:1181–88.
4. Dayer J-M, Krane SM, Russell RGG, Robinson DR. Production of collagenase and prostaglandins by isolated adherent rheumatoid synovial cells. *Proc Natl Acad Sci USA.* 1976;73:945–9.

5. Mehindate K, Al-Daccak R, Dayer J-M, Kennedy BP, Kris C, Borgeat P et al. Superantigen-induced collagenase gene expression in human IFN-γ-treated fibroblast-like synoviocytes involves prostaglandin E_2. *J Immunol*. 1995;155:3570–7.

6. Ziche M, Jones J, Gullino PM. Role of prostaglandin E_1 and copper in angiogenesis. *J Natl Cancer Inst*. 1982;69:475–81.

7. Form DM, Auerbach R. PGE_2 and angiogenesis. *Proc Soc Exp Biol Med*. 1983;172:214–8.

8. Diaz-Flores L, Gutierrez R, Valladares F, Varela H, Perez M. Intense vascular sprouting from rat femoral vein induced by prostaglandins E_1 and E_2. *Anat Rec*. 1994;238:68–76.

9. Ben-Av P, Crofford LJ, Wilder RL, Hla T. Induction of vascular endothelial growth factor expression in synovial fibroblasts by prostaglandin E and interleukin-1: a potential mechanism for inflammatory angiogenesis. *FEBS Lett*. 1995;372:83–7.

10. Moilanen E. Prostanoids and leukotrienes in rheumatoid synovitis. *Pharmacol Toxicol*. 1994;75(suppl):4–8.

11. Weissmann G. Prostaglandins as modulators rather than mediators of inflammation. *J Lipid Mediat*. 1993;6:275–86.

12. Smith WL, DeWitt DL. Biochemistry of prostaglandin endoperoxide H synthase-1 and synthase-2 and their differential susceptibility to nonsteroidal anti-inflammatory drugs. *Semin Nephrol*. 1995;15:179–94.

13. Smith WL. Prostanoid biosynthesis and mechanisms of action. *Am J Physiol*. 1992;263:F181–F191.

14. Crofford LJ, Wilder RL, Ristimaki AP, Remmers EF, Epps HR, Hla T. Cyclooxygenase-1 and -2 expression in rheumatoid synovial tissues: effects of interleukin-1β, phorbol ester, and corticosteroids. *J Clin Invest*. 1994;93:1095–101.

15. Hulkower KI, Wertheimer SJ, Levin W, Coffey JW, Anderson CM, Chen T et al. Interleukin-1β induces cytosolic phospholipase A_2 and prostaglandin H synthase in rheumatoid synovial fibroblasts. Evidence for their roles in the production of prostaglandin E_2. *Arthritis Rheum*. 1994;37:653–61.

16. Ristimaki A, Garfinkel S, Wessendorf J, Maciag T, Hla T. Induction of cyclooxygenase-2 by interleukin-1 alpha. Evidence for post-transcriptional regulation. *J Biol Chem*. 1994;269:11769–75.

17. Geng Y, Blance FJ, Cornelisson M, Lotz M. Regulation of cyclooxygenase-2 expression in normal human articular chondrocytes. *J Immunol*. 1995;155:796–801.

18. de Brum-Fernandes AJ, Laporte S, Heroux M, Lora M, Patry C, Menard HA et al. Expression of prostaglandin endoperoxide synthase-1 and prostaglandin endoperoxide synthase-2 in human osteoblasts. *Biochem Biophys Res Commun*. 1994;198:955–60.

19. Onoe Y, Miyaura C, Kaminakayashiki T, Nagai Y, Noguchi K, Chen Q-R et al. IL-13 and IL-4 inhibit bone resorption by suppressing cyclooxygenase-2-dependent prostaglandin synthesis in osteoblasts. *J Immunol*. 1996;156:758–64.

20. Hempel SL, Monick MM, He B, Yano T, Hunninghake GW. Synthesis of prostaglandin H synthase-2 by human alveolar macrophages in response to lipopolysaccharide is inhibited by decreased cell oxidant tone. *J Biol Chem*. 1994;269:32979–84.

21. Arias-Negrete S, Keller K, Chadee K. Proinflammatory cytokines regulated cyclooxygenase-2 mRNA expression in human macrophages. *Biochem Biophys Res Commun*. 1995;208:582–9.

22. Appleby SB, Ristimaki A, Neilson K, Narko K, Hla T. Structure of the human cyclooxygenase-2 gene. *Biochem J*. 1994;302:723–7.

23. Crofford LJ, Tan B, McCarthy CJ, Hla T. NF-κB is involved in the regulation of cyclooxygenase-2 expression by interleukin-1β in rheumatoid synoviocytes. *Arthritis Rheum*. 1997;40:226–36.

24. Yamaoka K, Otsuka T, Niiro H, Arinobu, Y, Niho, Y, Hamasaki, N et al. Activation of STAT5 by lipopolysaccharide through granulocyte-macrophage colony-stimulating factor production in human monocytes. *J Immunol*. 1998;160:838–45.
25. Xie W, Herschman HR. Transcriptional regulation of prostaglandin synthase 2 gene expression by platelet-derived growth factor and serum. *J Biol Chem*. 1996;271:31742–8.
26. Zhang Y, Cao HJ, Graf B, Meekings H, Smith TJ, Phipps RP. CD40 engagement up-regulates cyclooxygenase-2 expression and prostaglandin E_2 production in human lung fibroblasts. *J Immunol*. 1998;160:1053–7.
27. Rissoan MC, Van Kooten C, Chomarat P, Galibert L, Durand I, Thivolet-Bejui F et al. The functional CD40 antigen of fibroblasts may contribute to the proliferation of rheumatoid synovium. *Clin Exp Immunol*. 1996;106:481–90.
28. Anderson GD, Hauser SD, Bremer ME, McGarity KL, Isakson PC, Gregory SA. Selective inhibition of cyclooxygenase-2 reverses inflammation and expression of COX-2 and IL-6 in rat adjuvant arthritis. *J Clin Invest*. 1996;97:2672–79.
29. Masferrer JL, Zweifel BS, Seibert K, Needleman P. Selective regulation of cellular cyclooxygenase by dexamethasone and endotoxin in mice. *J Clin Invest*. 1990;86:1375–9.
30. Masferrer JL, Seibert K, Zweifel B, Needleman P. Endogenous glucocorticoids regulate an inducible cyclooxygenase enzyme. *Proc Natl Acad Sci USA*. 1992;89:3917–21.
31. Sano H, Hla T, Maier JAM, Crofford LJ, Case JP, Maciag T et al. In vivo cyclooxygenase expression in synovial tissues of patients with rheumatoid arthritis and osteoarthritis and rats with adjuvant and streptococcal cell wall arthritis. *J Clin Invest*. 1992;89:97–108.
32. DeWitt DL, Meade EA. Serum and glucocorticoid regulation of gene transcription and expression of the prostaglandin H synthase-1 and prostaglandin H synthase-2 isozymes. *Arch Biochem Biophys*. 1993;306:94–102.
33. Siegle I, Klein T, Backman JT, Saal JG, Nüsing RM, Fritz P. Expression of cyclooxygenase 1 and cyclooxygenase 2 in human synovial tissue. Differential elevation of cyclooxygenase 2 in inflammatory joint diseases. *Arthritis Rheum*. 1998;41:122–9.
34. Futaki N, Takahashi S, Yokoyama M, Arai I, Higuchi S, Otomo S. NS-398, a new anti-inflammatory agent, selectively inhibits prostaglandin G/H synthase/cyclooxygenase (COX-2) activity in vitro. *Prostaglandins*. 1994;47:55–9.
35. Wery JP, Schevitz RW, Clawson DK, Bobbitt JL, Dow ER, Gamboa G et al. Structure of recombinant human rheumatoid arthritic synovial fluid phospholipase A_2 at 2.2 Å resolution. *Nature*. 1991;352:79–82.

Cyclooxygenase-2 and bone resorption

C. C. PILBEAM

Bone is a dynamic tissue that is undergoing continuous turnover, cycles of resorption and formation, throughout life. This remodelling occurs in discrete pockets throughout the skeleton. The process begins with the removal of the unmineralized matrix material that appears to prevent resorption and the arrival of osteoclasts, which then resorb the mineralized matrix. Osteoclasts are large multinucleated cells arising through a process of proliferation and differentiation from haematopoietic mononuclear cells in the bone marrow. Factors that stimulate formation of osteoclasts are thought to do so by acting on marrow stromal cells, a group of supporting cells which include osteoblasts and which are descended from a common mesenchymal stem cell. These cells then produce paracrine factors, such as macrophage colony stimulating factor, which are necessary for osteoclastic differentiation. In addition, physical contact between osteoclastic and osteoblastic precursors is necessary for the generation of active osteoclasts. Following the completion of resorption, osteoblasts produce new bone matrix. Resorption is said to be 'coupled' to formation in that resorption is followed by formation as long as the template for formation is preserved. The identity of these coupling factors is unknown. They may be factors released from the bone matrix during resorption, such as transforming growth factor (TGF)-β, or factors produced by osteoblastic or marrow stromal cells, such as prostaglandins (PGs). Imbalance in this cycle, such as occurs on oestrogen withdrawal when resorption is accelerated more than formation, can lead to bone loss and bone fracture.

PATHOLOGICAL ROLES FOR COX-2 IN BONE

Non-steroidal anti-inflammatory drugs (NSAIDs) are commonly prescribed to control inflammation and pain. Because of the differential expression and regulation of cyclooxygenase-1 and -2 (COX-1 and -2), it has been postulated that COX-2 is the major synthase involved in inflammatory responses, while COX-1 produces prostanoids needed for ongoing 'housekeeping' functions, such as maintenance of renal blood flow, platelet aggregation and gastric cytoprotection. This has led to the development of highly selective inhibitors of COX-2 activity, which are predicted to have better anti-inflammatory actions than older NSAIDs and to cause less gastric pathology. In support of this hypothesis, a number of studies have reported that PG production is increased in inflammatory processes. Because of the association of PG production with inflammation and because PGs are potent stimulators of bone resorption, it is often assumed that PGs are responsible for some of the bone loss and cartilage destruction associated with inflammatory diseases. However, there are only a few studies which have shown that inhibiting PG production can influence bone loss, such as those showing that NSAIDs can decrease alveolar bone loss in periodontitis[1-3].

There is a possible role for COX-2 in tumourigenesis in some tissues. Overexpression of COX-2 is implicated as an early abnormality in colon carcinoma, and inhibition of COX-2 activity can suppress growth of tumours in animal models[4]. The effects are probably not specific for COX-2 since programmed overexpression of COX-1 has also been associated with tumourigenesis[5], and both COX-1 and -2 overexpression is found in other cancers[6]. We have screened several osteoblastic cell lines derived from human osteosarcomas and not found overexpression of either COX. In MG-63 cells, COX-1 is constitutively expressed and COX-2 is inducible[7]. Preliminary studies suggest that G292 cells are similar to MG63 cells, while SaOs cells may not express COX-2 at all (data not shown). On the other hand, ROS 17/2.8 cells, a rat osteosarcoma cell line, express the highest levels of COX-1 mRNA of any osteoblastic cell that we have studied, and we cannot induce COX-2 in these cells[8]. Hence, abnormal expression of COX may be one of several factors characterizing osteosarcomas but does not appear critical to their aetiology.

ROLE OF COX-2 IN BONE TURNOVER

Regulation of COX-2 Expression in Osteoblasts

PGs are abundant in bone. Osteoblasts produce PGs and express PG receptors[9]. PG receptors have not been demonstrated in osteoclasts, and it is assumed that the PGs produced in co-cultures of osteoblasts and osteoclasts are made by osteoblasts. However, because it is not yet possible to identify osteoclastic precursor cells, they may produce PGs as well as respond to them.

The regulation of PG production in bone occurs largely via regulation of COX-2 expression and this regulation is generally transcriptional[9]. COX-2 expression is usually low or undetectable in unstimulated osteoblasts but can be rapidly induced by many regulators of bone metabolism, while COX-1 is constitutively expressed. COX-2 agonists include cytokines [interleukin (IL)-1, IL-6 and tumour necrosis factor (TNF)-α], growth factors [fibroblast growth factor (FGF)-2, TGF-β and TGF-α] and parathyroid hormone (PTH)[10–17]. Exogenous and endogenous PGs also induce COX-2 and can, therefore, amplify PG responses[12,18]. Fluid shear stress, thought to be the means by which mechanical loads are transduced to bone cells, induces COX-2 expression and PG production in cultured osteoblastic cells[19]. There are fewer inhibitors of COX-2 expression in bone. Glucocorticoids are potent inhibitors of stimulated COX-2 mRNA and protein expression in osteoblasts[10,12]. We have shown that retinoic acid can transcriptionally inhibit the induction of COX-2 expression by a broad variety of agonists[20]. IL-4 and IL-13 also inhibit COX-2 expression and PG production in bone organ and cell cultures[14,21].

Effects of PGs on Bone Formation In Vitro
The effects of exogenous PGs on bone formation in vitro are complex. PGs can stimulate DNA synthesis and cell replication in bone cell and organ cultures[22]. In organ culture the mitogenic effect of PGE_2 appears to be selective for pre-osteoblasts[23]. Exposure time and dose may be important. In periosteal cells from embryonic chick calvariae, the mitogenic effect of PGE_2 is greatest after brief exposure and decreases with prolonged exposure[24]. A dose-related biphasic effect has been reported in cultured human bone cells with stimulation of mitogenesis at 10^{-9}M PGE_2 and inhibition at 10^{-6}M[25]. In marrow stromal cell and primary calvarial cell cultures designed to study differentiation of osteoblasts from progenitors, PGE_2 stimulates the formation of colony forming units and mineralized nodules[26–28]. PGs can both stimulate and inhibit the synthesis of collagen, the major bone matrix protein[9]. The inhibitory effect appears to be a transcriptional effect on the collagen promoter[29]. Hence, PGs enhance the proliferation and differentiation of pre-osteoblasts but can inhibit the production of collagen by mature osteoblasts.

Effects of PGs on Bone Formation In Vivo
In vivo, many animal experiments have shown that prolonged systemic administration of PGE_2 stimulates both endosteal and periosteal new bone formation[30]. In addition, PGE_2 given in vivo enhances osteoblastic differentiation in explanted marrow stromal cells[31]. Little is known about the role of endogenous PGs in vivo. Mechanical loading stimulates PG production in bone cells, and the increased bone formation that occurs after mechanical loading in animals can be blocked by NSAIDs[32,33], suggesting that endogenous PGs also stimulate bone formation.

Effects of PGs on Bone Resorption
PGs, especially PGs of the E series, are potent stimulators of resorption in cultured neonatal calvariae or foetal long bones from rodents[9]. Many factors that stimulate PG production also stimulate resorption in organ culture systems, and the stimulated resorption is sometimes shown to be mediated in part by PG production. However, data on the PG-dependence of stimulated resorption are

variable and often contradictory. For example, IL-1, a potent stimulator of PG production, has both PG-dependent[34] and PG-independent[35] effects on bone resorption. Boyce et al.[36] showed that injection of IL-1 above the calvariae of mice causes an initial short-term PG-independent stimulation of bone resorption, followed by a sustained PG-dependent stimulation of bone resorption. Indomethacin partially inhibits FGF-2-mediated resorption in organ culture[13]. Although PTH is a potent stimulator of PG production, PTH-stimulated resorption in organ culture is not inhibited by NSAIDs[14]. Inhibition of resorption by IL-4, an inhibitor of COX-2 expression, is reported to be both PG-dependent[21] and PG-independent[14]. TGFα-stimulated resorption is reported to be PG-dependent in calvariae but PG-independent in foetal long bones[37].

Effects of PGs on Osteoclastogenesis

PGE_1 and PGE_2, but not $PGF_{2\alpha}$, stimulate osteoclast formation in bone marrow cultures[38,39]. In contrast to the results in organ culture, studies in marrow culture consistently find that stimulation of osteoclast formation is dependent on PG production. Agonists that have been reported to stimulate PG-dependent osteoclastogenesis include IL-1[34,40], TNF-α[40], PTH[41,42], 1,25(OH)$_2$ vitamin D[43], IL-11[44], IL-6[17], phorbol ester[45] and FGF-2[46].

Formation of bone-resorbing osteoclasts requires a contact-dependent interaction between haematopoietic osteoclast precursor cells and stromal or osteoblastic cells[47,48]. This interaction is postulated to occur via an osteoclast differentiating factor (ODF), which has recently been identified as a molecule made by stromal cells and osteoblasts that binds osteoprotegerin (OPG) and is, therefore, also called OPG ligand (OPGL)[49,50]. ODF or OPGL is a TNF-related cytokine and is identical to the molecule previously called TRANCE or RANKL and found on T cells. OPG, which inhibits bone resorption and is also called osteoclastogenesis inhibitory factor, is a soluble member of the TNF receptor family[51]. PGE_2 can induce expression of ODF/OPGL mRNA[49], and inhibition of ODF/OPGL blocks PGE_2-stimulated resorption[52]. Both haematopoietic precursors and stromal cells are present in bone marrow culture systems, but osteoclast progenitor cells devoid of stromal cells can be obtained from the spleen. PGE_2 can stimulate the formation of osteoclast precursors, positive for calcitonin receptors, in cultures of spleen cells but these cells will not resorb bone unless they interact with stromal cells[43].

Hence, it seems likely that PGs may act at early stages of osteoclast differentiation, prior to the interaction with stromal cells which is necessary to produce activated osteoclasts. Studies showing that activation of mature osteoclasts in vitro is not dependent on PGs and, in fact, that PGs can transiently inhibit bone resorption when added to isolated mature osteoclasts in vitro, support this suggestion[53]. If PGs have their major effect on differentiation of osteoclast precursors, then the variability in, or lack of, PG-dependent resorption in organ culture may be explained if resorption in organ culture depends heavily on activation of, rather than formation of, osteoclasts.

SUMMARY

The actions of PGs on skeletal metabolism are complex, and the role of PGs in vivo is still unclear. The new selective inhibitors of COX-2 should help to clarify the endogenous role of COX-2 in bone metabolism. In vitro studies with currently available NSAIDs indicate that they can have biphasic effects; that is, low concentrations can increase, rather than decrease, PG production[54,55]. Hence, to obtain a consistent inhibitory effect of NSAIDs in vivo, frequent administration and high doses are necessary, and this may produce toxicity. The new COX-2-selective inhibitors, which have less gastric toxicity and less effect on platelet aggregation, can be administered at higher doses. Moreover, the increased COX activity at low NSAID dose may be the result of the substrate-dependent, positive cooperative activation of COX-1 which is only seen with non-selective NSAIDs[56].

As the synthase responsible for acute PG responses to multiple physiological and pathological agents considered important in skeletal metabolism, it seems likely that the role of COX-2 in bone is much more than simply mediation of inflammation. We speculate that whether effects are catabolic or anabolic in general will depend on the amplitude and duration of the COX-2 response, as well as on the current state of remodelling. From studies of resorption in organ culture systems and in vivo, it is clear that inflammatory agents, such as IL-1, can stimulate bone resorption independently of PG production. However, the ability to maintain prolonged resorption may depend on PGs, and, hence, inhibition of COX-2 may decrease bone resorption. The inhibitory effect of PGs on isolated osteoclast activity is thought to be transient and hence of lesser importance than the stimulatory effects. On the other hand, if PGs couple the inflammation-stimulated resorptive responses to bone formation, then potent inhibitors of COX-2 may eventually lead to decreased anabolic responses and increased bone loss.

REFERENCES

1. Howell TH, Jeffcoat MK, Goldhaber P, Reddy MS, Kaplan ML, Johnson HG et al. Inhibition of alveolar bone loss in beagles with the NSAID naproxen. *J Periodontal Res*. 1991;26:498–501.
2. Jeffcoat MK, Reddy MS, Moreland LW, Koopman WJ. Effects of nonsteroidal anti-inflammatory drugs on bone loss in chronic inflammatory disease. *Ann N Y Acad Sci*. 1993;696:292–302.
3. Cavanaugh PFJ, Meredith MP, Buchanan W, Doyle MJ, Reddy MS, Jeffcoat MK. Coordinate production of PGE$_2$ and IL-1β in the gingival crevicular fluid of adults with periodontitis: its relationship to alveolar bone loss and disruption by twice daily treatment with ketorolac tromethamine oral rinse. *J Periodontal Res*. 1998;33:75–82.
4. Williams CS, Luongo C, Radhika A, Zhang T, Lamps LW, Nanney LB et al. Elevated cyclooxygenase-2 levels in *Min* mouse adenomas. *Gastroenterology*. 1996;111:1134–40.
5. Narko K, Ristimäki A, MacPhee M, Smith E, Haudenschild CC, Hla T. Tumorigenic transformation of immortalized ECV endothelial cells by cyclooxygenase-1 overexpression. *J Biol Chem*. 1997;272:21455–60.

6. Hwang D, Scollard D, Byrne J, Levine E. Expression of cyclooxygenase-1 and cyclo-oxygenase-2 in human breast cancer. *J Natl Cancer Inst.* 1998;90:455–60.

7. Min Y-K, Rao Y, Okada Y, Raisz LG, Pilbeam CC. Regulation of prostaglandin G/H synthase-2 expression by interleukin-1 in human osteoblast-like cells. *J Bone Miner Res.* 1998;13:1066–75.

8. Pilbeam CC, Fall PM, Alander CB, Raisz LG. Differential effects of nonsteroidal anti-inflammatory drugs on constitutive and inducible prostaglandin G/H synthase in cultured bone cells. *J Bone Miner Res.* 1997;12:1198–203.

9. Pilbeam CC, Harrison JR, Raisz LG. Prostaglandins and bone metabolism. In: Bilezikian JP, Raisz LG, Rodan GA editors. *Principles of Bone Biology.* New York: Academic Press; 1996:715–28.

10. Pilbeam CC, Kawaguchi H, Hakeda Y, Voznesensky O, Alander CB, Raisz LG. Differential regulation of inducible and constitutive prostaglandin endoperoxide synthase in osteo-blastic MC3T3-E1 cells. *J Biol Chem.* 1993;268:25643–9.

11. Harrison JR, Lorenzo JA, Kawaguchi H, Raisz LG, Pilbeam CC. Stimulation of prostaglandin E_2 production by interleukin-1 and transforming growth factor-α in osteoblastic MC3T3-E1 cells. *J Bone Miner Res.* 1994;9:817–23.

12. Kawaguchi H, Raisz LG, Voznesensky OS, Alander CB, Hakeda Y, Pilbeam CC. Regulation of the two prostaglandin G/H synthases by parathyroid hormone, interleukin-1, cortisol and prostaglandin E_2 in cultured neonatal mouse calvariae. *Endocrinology.* 1994;135:1157–64.

13. Kawaguchi H, Pilbeam CC, Gronowicz G, Abreu C, Fletcher BS, Herschman HR et al. Regulation of inducible prostaglandin G/H synthase mRNA levels and promoter activity by basic fibroblast growth factor in osteoblastic cells. *J Clin Invest.* 1995;96:923–30.

14. Kawaguchi H, Nemoto K, Raisz LG, Harrison JR, Voznesensky OS, Alander CB et al. Interleukin-4 inhibits prostaglandin G/H synthase-2 and cytosolic phospholipase A_2 induction in neonatal mouse parietal bone cultures. *J Bone Miner Res.* 1996;11:358–66.

15. Tetradis S, Pilbeam CC, Liu Y, Herschman HR, Kream BE. Parathyroid hormone increases prostaglandin G/H synthase-2 transcription by a cyclic adenosine 3′,5′-monophosphate-mediated pathway in murine osteoblastic MC3T3-E1 cells. *Endocrinology.* 1997;138:3594–600.

16. Pilbeam CC, Rao Y, Voznesensky O, Kawaguchi H, Alander C, Raisz LG et al. Transforming growth factor-β1 regulation of prostaglandin G/H synthase-2 expression in osteoblastic MC3T3-E1 cells. *Endocrinology.* 1997;138:4672–82.

17. Tai H, Miyaura C, Pilbeam CC, Tamura T, Ohsugi Y, Koishihara Y et al. Transcriptional induction of cyclooxygenase-2 in osteoblasts is involved in interleukin-6-induced osteoclast formation. *Endocrinology.* 1997;138:2372–9.

18. Pilbeam CC, Raisz LG, Voznesensky O, Alander CB, Delman BN, Kawaguchi K. Autoregulation of inducible prostaglandin G/H synthase in osteoblastic cells by prostaglandins. *J Bone Miner Res.* 1994;10:406–14.

19. Klein-Nulend J, Burger EH, Semeins CM, Raisz LG, Pilbeam CC. Pulsating fluid flow stimulates prostaglandin release and inducible prostaglandin G/H synthase mRNA expression in primary mouse bone cells. *J Bone Miner Res.* 1997;12:45–51.

20. Pilbeam C, Bernecker P, Harrison J, Alander C, Voznesensky O, Herschman H et al. Retinoic acid inhibits induction of prostaglandin G/H synthase-2 mRNA and promoter activity in MC3T3-E1 osteoblastic cells. *J Bone Miner Res.* 1995;10(suppl 1):S496.

21. Onoe Y, Miyaura C, Kaminakayashiki T, Nagai Y, Noguchi K, Chen QR et al. IL-13 and IL-4 inhibit bone resorption by suppressing cyclooxygenase-2- dependent prostaglandin synthesis in osteoblasts. *J Immunol.* 1996;156:758–64.

22. Woodiel FN, Fall PM, Raisz LG. Anabolic effects of prostaglandins in cultured fetal rat calvariae: structure–activity relations and signal transduction pathway. *J Bone Miner Res.* 1996;11:1249–55.

23. Gronowicz GA, Fall PM, Raisz LG. Prostaglandin E$_2$ stimulates preosteoblast replication: an autoradiographic study in cultured fetal rat calvariae. *Exp Cell Res.* 1994;212:314–20.

24. Scutt A, Duvos C, Lauber J, Mayer H. Time-dependent effects of parathyroid hormone and prostaglandin E$_2$ on DNA synthesis by periosteal cells from embryonic chick calvaria. *Calcif Tissue Int.* 1994;55:208–15.

25. Baylink TM, Mohan S, Fitzsimmons RJ, Baylink DJ. Evaluation of signal transduction mechanisms for the mitogenic effects of prostaglandin E$_2$ in normal human bone cells in vitro. *J Bone Miner Res.* 1996;11:1413–8.

26. Flanagan AM, Chambers TJ. Stimulation of bone nodule formation *in vitro* by prostaglandins E$_1$ and E$_2$. *Endocrinology.* 1992;130:443–8.

27. Nagata T, Kaho K, Nishikawa S, Shinohara H, Wakano Y, Ishida H. Effect of prostaglandin E$_2$ on mineralization of bone nodules formed by fetal rat calvarial cells. *Calcif Tissue Int.* 1994;55:451–7.

28. Scutt A, Bertram P. Bone marrow cells are targets for the anabolic actions of prostaglandin E$_2$ on bone: induction of a transition from nonadherent to adherent osteoblast precursors. *J Bone Miner Res.* 1995;10:474–87.

29. Fall PM, Breault DT, Raisz LG. Inhibition of collagen synthesis by prostaglandins in the immortalized rat osteoblastic cell line, Py1a: structure activity relations and signal transduction mechanisms. *J Bone Miner Res.* 1994;9:1935–43.

30. Jee WS, Ma YF. The in vivo anabolic actions of prostaglandins in bone. *Bone.* 1997;21:297-304.

31. Weinreb M, Suponitzky I, Keila S. Systemic administration of an anabolic dose of PGE$_2$ in young rats increases the osteogenic capacity of bone marrow. *Bone.* 1997;20:521–6.

32. Pead MJ, Lanyon LE. Indomethacin modulation of load-related stimulation of new bone formation in vivo. *Calcif Tissue Int.* 1989;45:34–40.

33. Chow JW, Chambers TJ. Indomethacin has distinct early and late actions on bone formation induced by mechanical stimulation. *Am J Physiol.* 1994;267:E287–E292.

34. Akatsu T, Takahashi N, Udagawa N, Imamura K, Yamaguchi A, Sato K et al. Role of prostaglandins in interleukin-1-induced bone resorption in mice in vitro. *J Bone Miner Res.* 1991;6:183–9.

35. Garrett IR, Mundy GR. Relationship between interleukin-1 and prostaglandins in resorbing neonatal calvaria. *J Bone Miner Res.* 1989;4:789–94.

36. Boyce BF, Aufdemorte TB, Garrett IR, Yates AJP, Mundy GR. Effects of interleukin-1 on bone turnover in normal mice. *Endocrinology.* 1989;125:1142–50.

37. Stern PH, Krieger NS, Nissenson RA, Williams RD, Winkler ME, Derynck R et al. Human transforming growth factor-alpha stimulates bone resorption in vitro. *J Clin Invest.* 1985;76:2016–9.

38. Collins DA, Chambers TJ. Effect of prostaglandins E$_1$, E$_2$, and F$_{2\alpha}$ on osteoclast formation in mouse bone marrow cultures. *J Bone Miner Res.* 1991;6:157–64.

39. Kaji H, Sugimoto T, Kanatani M, Fukase M, Kumegawa M, Chihara K. Prostaglandin E$_2$ stimulates osteoclast-like cell formation and bone resorbing activity via osteoblasts: role of cAMP-dependent protein kinase. *J Bone Miner Res.* 1996;11:62–71.

40. Lader CS, Flanagan AM. Prostaglandin E$_2$, interleukin 1α, and tumor necrosis factor-α increase human osteoclast formation and bone resorption in vitro. *Endocrinology.* 1998;139:3157–64.

41. Inoue H, Tanaka N, Uchiyama C. Parathyroid hormone increases the number of tartrate-resistant acid phosphatase-positive cells through prostaglandin E$_2$ synthesis in adherent cell culture of neonatal rat bones. *Endocrinology.* 1995;136:3648–56.

42. Sato T, Morita I, Murota S. Prostaglandin E$_2$ mediates parathyroid hormone induced osteoclast formation by cyclic AMP independent mechanism. *Adv Exp Med Biol.* 1997;407:383–6.

43. Collins DA, Chambers TJ. Prostaglandin E_2 promotes osteoclast formation in murine hematopoietic cultures through an action on hematopoietic cells. *J Bone Miner Res.* 1992;7:555–61.

44. Girasole G, Passeri G, Jilka RL, Manolagas SC. Interleukin-11: a new cytokine critical for osteoclast development. *J Clin Invest.* 1994;93:1516–24.

45. Amano S, Hanazawa S, Kawata Y, Nakada Y, Miyata Y, Kitano S. Phorbol myristate acetate stimulates osteoclast formation in 1α,25-dihydroxyvitamin D_3-primed mouse embryonic calvarial cells by a prostaglandin-dependent mechanism. *J Bone Miner Res.* 1994;9:465–72.

46. Hurley MM, Lee SK, Raisz LG, Bernecker P, Lorenzo J. Basic fibroblast growth factor induces osteoclast formation in murine bone marrow cultures. *Bone.* 1998;22:309–16.

47. Thomson BM, Saklatvala J, Chambers TJ. Osteoblasts mediate interleukin 1 stimulation of bone resorption by rat osteoclasts. *J Exp Med.* 1986;164:104–12.

48. Jimi E, Nakamura I, Amano H, Taguchi Y, Tsurukai T, Tamura M et al. Osteoclast function is activated by osteoblastic cells through a mechanism involving cell-to-cell contact. *Endocrinology.* 1996;137:2187–90.

49. Yasuda H, Shima N, Nakagawa N, Yamaguchi K, Kinosaki M, Mochizuki S et al. Osteoclast differentiation factor is a ligand for osteoprotegerin/osteoclastogenesis-inhibitory factor and is identical to TRANCE/RANKL. *Proc Natl Acad Sci USA.* 1998;95:3597–602.

50. Lacey DL, Timms E, Tan HL, Kelley MJ, Dunstan CR, Burgess T et al. Osteoprotegerin ligand is a cytokine that regulates osteoclast differentiation and activation. *Cell.* 1998;93:165–76.

51. Yasuda H, Shima N, Nakagawa N, Mochizuki SI, Yano K, Fujise N et al. Identity of osteoclastogenesis inhibitory factor (OCIF) and osteoprotegerin (OPG): a mechanism by which OPG/OCIF inhibits osteoclastogenesis in vitro. *Endocrinology.* 1998;139:1329–37.

52. Tsukii K, Shima N, Mochizuki S, Yamaguchi K, Kinosaki M, Yano K et al. Osteoclast differentiation factor mediates an essential signal for bone resorption induced by 1α,25-dihydroxyvitamin D_3, prostaglandin E_2, or parathyroid hormone in the microenvironment of bone. *Biochem Biophys Res Commun.* 1998;246:337–41.

53. Chambers TJ, McSheehy PM, Thomson BM, Fuller K. The effect of calcium-regulating hormones and prostaglandins on bone resorption by osteoclasts disaggregated from neonatal rabbit bones. *Endocrinology.* 1985;116:234–9.

54. Raisz LG, Simmons HA, Fall PM. Biphasic effects of nonsteroidal anti-inflammatory drugs on prostaglandin production by cultured rat calvariae. *Prostaglandins.* 1989;37:559–65.

55. Lindsley HB, Smith DD. Enhanced prostaglandin E_2 secretion by cytokine-stimulated human synoviocytes in the presence of subtherapeutic concentrations of nonsteroidal antiinflammatory drugs. *Arthritis Rheum.* 1990;33:1162–9.

56. Swinney DC, Mak AY, Barnett J, Ramesha CS. Differential allosteric regulation of prostaglandin H synthase 1 and 2 by arachidonic acid. *J Biol Chem.* 1997;272:12393–8.

6

The clinical epidemiology of non-steroidal anti-inflammatory drug gastropathy

J. F. FRIES, G. SINGH AND D. R. RAMEY

The gastropathy associated with non-steroidal anti-inflammatory drug (NSAID) use has become recognized as the most damaging set of side effects from any class of therapeutic agents. NSAID gastropathy results from depletion of prostaglandins from the gastrointestinal (GI) mucosa, particularly in the stomach but also in other parts of the GI tract. Prostaglandin depletion can lead to development of silent ulcers with consequent haemorrhage, perforation or other complications. NSAID side effects of nausea, epigastric pain and other GI symptoms are largely, if not entirely, due to other effects of the drugs and do not correlate well with serious events which result in hospitalization or death. It is the serious events and not the symptoms or the endoscopic ulcers which constitute this modern epidemic. ARAMIS (Arthritis, Rheumatism and Aging Medical Information System) has made substantial contributions to our understanding of the clinical epidemiology of this condition and our knowledge of ways to reduce the magnitude of the epidemic[1].

ARAMIS is the national arthritis data resource, containing longitudinal outcome data with rigorous follow up on 36,000 patients with rheumatic disease from 17 centres in the US and Canada, studied over nearly 100,000 patient-years. Information on long-term aspects of treatment and prognosis has been recorded prospectively at six-month intervals over the past 20 years with regard to use of NSAIDs and other classes of drugs used in the management of the rheumatic diseases. Outcomes are expressed in terms of the '5Ds' of outcome (death, disability, discomfort, drug toxicity and destitution)[2]. ARAMIS scales, instruments and protocols have been extensively validated and have resulted in over 900 peer-reviewed publications.

Until recently, post-marketing surveillance programmes were concerned mainly with the reporting of adverse drug reactions. However, prospective longitudinal databases, such as ARAMIS, allow a more complete study of outcomes for patients with rheumatic disease[3]. With the assistance of ARAMIS data sets it is possible to address the following questions which cannot, by definition, be addressed prior to the marketing of a drug. (1) What is the incidence of serious NSAID gastropathy events in rheumatoid arthritis (RA) and osteoarthritis (OA)? (2) What are the US and international totals for hospitalization and deaths from this cause? (3) How do these compare with numbers of deaths from other diseases? (4) Which variables predict high risk for particular individuals? (5) What predictive models can be developed to identify individuals at high risk? (6) What are the differences, if any, in serious toxic events between different NSAIDs?

With the ARAMIS data banks, we have sought not to identify rare side effects, but rather to address the common, and clinically most important, side effects which account for the great majority of drug-caused morbidity and mortality[3-5].

HOSPITALIZATIONS AND DEATHS ASSOCIATED WITH NSAID THERAPY FOR RA AND OA

GI complications in OA and RA are summarized in Table 1. This prospective study of 2921 patients with RA and 1283 patients with OA included over 15,000 patient-years of observation, the majority of which represented exposure to NSAIDs. GI events requiring hospitalization were observed in 134 RA patients and 19 OA

Table 1 Gastrointestinal complications in RA and OA

	RA (n = 2921)		OA (n = 1283)
	Hospitalizations	Deaths	Hospitalizations
Person-years of observation	12,224	12,224	3234
Person-years taking NSAIDs	8471	8471	2199
Person-years not taking NSAIDs	3753	3753	1035
GI events (number)	134	26	19
GI events on NSAIDs (number)	124	19	16
Rate per year on NSAIDs (%)	1.46 (S.E. 0.13)[a]	0.22	0.73 (S.E. 0.18)[a]
GI events not on NSAIDs (number)	10	2	3
Rate per year not on NSAIDS (%)	0.27	0.05	0.29
Relative risk on NSAIDs	5.49	4.21	2.51
Excess rate on NSAIDs	1.19	0.17	0.44
Upper GI hospitalizations (number)	108	—	11
Upper GI hospitalizations per year on NSAIDs (%)	1.27	—	0.50
Lower GI hospitalizations (number)	16	—	5
Lower GI hospitalizations per year on NSAIDs (%)	0.19	—	0.23

[a]RA vs OA (P<0.001)

patients; over 90% of these events occurred while patients were taking NSAIDs. The rate of GI hospitalizations per year for those taking NSAIDs was 1.46% in RA and exactly half of that in OA. The relative risk for these patients while on NSAIDs was 5.49 times the risk while not on NSAIDs in RA and 2.51 times the risk in OA. Subtracting the background frequency, the excess rate while on NSAIDs is about 1.2% per year in RA and approximately 0.44% per year in OA. Upper GI hospitalizations strongly predominate over lower GI hospitalizations, but relative risks for lower GI complications are similar between the two groups[1,6].

There were 26 deaths from serious NSAID gastropathy events in RA patients of whom 19 were definitely known to have taken NSAIDs. The relative risk of GI death for those on NSAIDs versus those not on NSAIDs is thus over 4.2 and the excess rate of death is nearly 2 per 1000 per year, or 0.2%.

NATIONAL AND INTERNATIONAL INCIDENCE

Estimates of the incidence of NSAIDs-associated GI hospitalizations and deaths in the US are provided in Table 2[7]. Death rates were estimated from the data given above and from the expected ratio of excess GI deaths to GI hospitalizations (approximately 1 in 10). About 107,000 hospitalizations occur each year in the US and approximately 16,500 deaths. These large numbers occur because of substantial, if not striking, risks for the individual patient and because of an extremely large number of patients exposed to these drugs.

Even more alarming data may be generated by estimating GI hospitalizations and deaths on an international basis and over the period since 1964 when NSAIDs began to be available (Table 3). These estimates assume US exposure at 50% of total international exposure, incidence rates to be similar across nations, and estimate exposure to NSAIDs over time from 1964 to 1997 to be 50% of 1997 exposure (since exposure was relatively light prior to 1975 or 1980). An estimated 260,000 hospitalizations occur worldwide each year, with approximately 26,000 deaths. Over the NSAID era since 1964, over four million hospitalizations and over 440,000 deaths are estimated to have occurred.

Table 2 NSAID-associated GI hospitalizations and deaths: national incidence estimates (US)

Diagnosis	Number of patients exposed (millions)	GI hospitalizations rate per year (%)	Number of hospitalizations per year (thousands)	GI death rate per year (%)[a]	Number of deaths per year (thousands)
RA	2	1.5	30	0.22	4.4
Probable RA	3	0.7	21	0.11	3.3
OA	8	0.7	56	0.11	8.8
Total	13		107		16.5

[a]Estimated from expected ratio of GI hospitalizations to excess GI deaths and from prospective data

Table 3 NSAID-associated GI hospitalizations and deaths: international incidence estimates

	Number of patient-years exposed (millions)	GI hospitalization rate per year (%)	Number of hospitalizations per year (thousands)	GI death rate per year (%)[c]	Number of deaths per year (thousands)
1997	26[a]	1.0	260	0.1	26
1964–1997	442[b]	1.0	4420	0.1	442[d]

[a]US exposure estimated at 50% of total international exposure. [b]Exposure numbers 1964–1997 (34 years) estimated at 50% of 1997 exposure. [c]Estimated from prospective data and ratio of GI deaths to GI hospitalizations (excess GI death rate). [d]Estimates exclude hospitalizations and deaths from aspirin, phenylbutazone, and other NSAIDs 1900–1964.

Figure 1 shows US death rates for several selected diseases. Death rates per 100,000 population due to NSAID-associated GI side effects are approximately twice those of asthma and malignant melanoma, and similar to those for all types of leukaemia combined. They are a significant fraction of deaths compared to diabetes or AIDS.

WHICH VARIABLES PREDICT SERIOUS GI ADVERSE EVENTS IN RA PATIENTS?

Table 4 compares those individuals experiencing serious GI events with those who did not, with regard to a number of variables. The strongest associations

Figure 1 Death rate per 100,000 and number of deaths from six selected causes, US population, 1994. Data from National Center for Health Statistics. GI complication rate based on ARAMIS data.

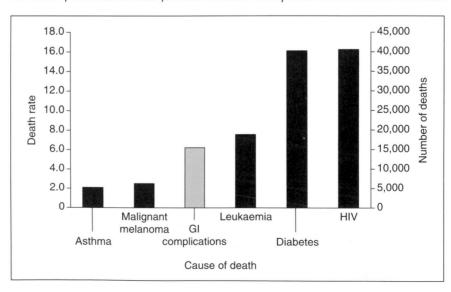

Table 4 Variables associated with GI hospitalization or death at predictive visit: RA patients

	GI events (n = 114)		No GI events (n = 1921)		
	Number	Mean (S.E.) or percent	Number	Mean (S.E.) or percent	P value
Age (years)	114	65.3 (1.0)	1921	59.6 (0.3)	<0.001
Education level (years)	112	12.0 (0.2)	1838	12.4 (0.1)	0.18
Disease duration (years)	113	19.2 (1.1)	1881	16.7 (0.2)	0.02
Disability index (0–3)	114	1.75 (0.07)	1921	1.38 (0.02)	<0.001
Smoking (packs/day)	37	0.2 (0.1)	1063	0.2 (0.01)	0.50
Alcohol (drinks/day)	82	0.4 (0.1)	1187	0.3 (0.02)	0.46
NSAID dose (% of maximum)	114	0.98 (0.05)	1921	0.86 (0.01)	0.013
Number of antacids or GI protective drugs	114	0.3 (0.05)	1921	0.2 (0.01)	0.08
Co-morbidity 1 [# of categories of non-rheumatic disease drugs taken] (0–8)	114	0.9 (0.1)	1921	0.6 (0.02)	0.008
Co-morbidity 2 [# of categories of non-rheumatic disease drugs taken ever] (0–8)	114	1.9 (0.1)	1921	1.4 (0.03)	0.0005
Female sex	114	72.8%	1921	76.3%	0.39
White race	114	94.7%	1921	92.0%	0.29
NSAID GI side effect ever	114	29.0%	1921	21.1%	0.05
Prednisone use	114	49.1%	1921	31.4%	<0.001
Antacids	91	15.4%	1744	8.5%	0.02
Co-morbidity 3 [Co-morbid condition reported ever]	114	84.2%	1921	75.7%	0.04

occur with older age, level of disability, presence of co-morbid conditions, prior NSAID GI side effects, use of oral prednisone, and use of antacids or H_2 antagonists[2,6]. Of interest, associations with education level, smoking, and alcohol were not significant; neither was female sex. Although three-quarters of events occur in women, exposure to these agents is also approximately three times greater in women than in men. Increased, rather than decreased, incidence in those taking antacids or H_2 antagonists has also been noted by other investigators. It appears that use of such agents reduces the level of minor symptoms, and increases the confidence of patients and physicians in the safety of the drugs, allowing longer use and higher dosage[8].

A MULTIVARIATE MODEL FOR PREDICTION OF RISK IN RA PATIENTS

A stepwise logistic regression which includes the variables of Table 4 is summarized in Table 5. The incidence of severe adverse events increases by 4% for each additional year of age over 50, nearly doubles with concurrent use of prednisone,

Table 5 Risk factors for GI complications (hospitalization or death) – stepwise logistic regression: RA patients

Variable	Coefficient (S.E.)	Odds ratio	95% Confidence interval for odds ratio
Age (year)	0.037 (0.01)	1.04	1.02–1.06
Prednisone (Y/N)	0.587 (0.20)	1.80	1.21–2.66
NSAID dose (% of max)	0.372 (0.17)	1.45	1.04–2.02
Disability (0–3)	0.287 (0.13)	1.33	1.03–1.72
Previous NSAID GI side effect (Y/N)	0.462 (0.22)	1.59	1.03–2.44

is associated with the dose of the NSAID, increases with disability level, and increases with previous reports of NSAID GI side effects. These five variables are sufficient to define most of the risk experienced by individual patients[6,8]. The major factor not included in this regression is the particular NSAID.

COMPARATIVE TOXICITY OF NSAIDS IN RA PATIENTS

Toxicity index scores incorporating GI symptoms and GI hospitalization are summarized in Table 6[4,6]. Selected NSAIDs are ranked in order of increasing GI toxicity. Differences of two- to three-fold exist between the drugs in the lower range of toxicity and those in the higher range. Preliminary data suggest that nabumetone and etodolac will eventually be placed toward the less toxic end of the range. Aspirin, long believed to be more toxic than the new NSAIDs, appears relatively non-toxic in these and other data. The striking difference between pre-marketing controlled trials of other NSAIDs against aspirin showing greater toxicity and the experience in the field showing less is largely due to differences

Table 6 GI toxicity index: RA patients

Drug	Number of patients	Toxicity index (Mean ± S.E.)
Salsalate	187	0.81 ± 0.51
Ibuprofen	577	1.13 ± 0.29
Aspirin	1521	1.18 ± 0.18
Sulindac	562	1.68 ± 0.29
Diclofenac	415	1.81 ± 0.35
Naproxen	1062	1.91 ± 0.21
Tolmetin	243	2.02 ± 0.44
Piroxicam	814	2.03 ± 0.24
Fenoprofen	158	2.35 ± 0.55
Indomethacin	418	2.39 ± 0.34
Ketoprofen	259	2.65 ± 0.43
Meclofenamate	165	3.91 ± 0.54

in dosage. In the pre-marketing trials, aspirin was employed in very high doses of 4–5 g per day. In practice, aspirin exposure is approximately one-half of this amount. In contrast, average NSAID doses have been gradually increased over the years and are now considerably higher than doses employed in the pre-marketing trials[9]. This phenomenon, explaining frequent differences between controlled trials and subsequent clinical experience, has been reported previously[9]. Other investigators have confirmed the two- to three-fold range of toxicity across different NSAIDs and have found very similar rank ordering of drugs, even though the 12 studies to date have used different methods, different patient populations and have been performed in different countries[10].

MANAGEMENT OF THE EPIDEMIC OF NSAID GASTROPATHY

The epidemic of NSAID gastropathy is a large one, neglected over time, and important to the public health. It is instructive to review the potential approaches to this epidemic. Initially, use of antacids and H_2 antagonists was felt to be a good approach, but these agents have been proven most likely to be harmful. Approaches such as taking NSAIDs with water or after meals are unstudied but are likely to produce the same problems. The pharmaceutical industry has responded to recognition of the NSAID gastropathy epidemic in several ways. One way has been to develop NSAIDs, such as nabumetone and etodolac, which it is hoped will be of lower toxicity. Another has been the development of synthetic prostaglandins, such as misoprostol, to counteract directly the causal mechanism of prostaglandin depletion. Misoprostol reduces the incidence of serious side effects by approximately 40 to 50%. This should be expected to make NSAIDs of medium toxicity such as naproxen, diclofenac, or piroxicam approximately as toxic as drugs at the safer end of the range such as ibuprofen or salsalate but at a potentially higher cost. This effect is not sufficiently strong to justify use of the most toxic NSAIDs unless there are strong clinical indications to the contrary in the individual patient. Probably the most important pharmacological advance will be the development and use of selective cyclo-oxygenase-2-inhibiting drugs, described extensively in the other articles in this volume[11]. These drugs promise to be important additions to our NSAID armamentarium.

Clinically, there have been other developments. In the management of RA there has been a shift in the recommended treatment strategy from one based upon NSAID use to one based on early and consistent use of disease modifying antirheumatic drugs[12]. As a result, many now recommend that NSAIDs be used only in lower doses and only as adjunctive symptomatic treatment for RA. This change should materially affect the magnitude of the NSAID gastropathy epidemic. In OA, emphasis has been placed on low doses of NSAIDs and use of acetaminophen whenever possible, rather than employing high dose NSAID treatment[13]. Exercise and other non-pharmacological modalities also are emphasized in the current approach to OA treatment. This change should also decrease the magnitude of the NSAID gastropathy epidemic. Clinically, at present, one should avoid NSAID use where less toxic therapy is of similar effectiveness, employ NSAIDs in lower doses whenever possible, and avoid the more toxic NSAIDs. In high risk patients who require potentially more toxic NSAIDs, addition of misoprostol may be indicated.

The arithmetic is straightforward. If NSAID use could be decreased by 50%, the magnitude of the epidemic should decrease by a similar amount. If lower doses were substituted for higher, another 50% reduction might be obtained. Use of the least toxic NSAIDs preferentially, including particularly the newer agents and those soon to come on the market, could result in a further 50% decrease resulting in only 12.5% of the current number of hospitalizations and deaths. This is a treatable epidemic.

SUMMARY

NSAID gastropathy is a serious but preventable problem. The contributions of clinical epidemiology to clinical practice are well supported by the studies in this area. The epidemiologist seeks first to quantify the magnitude of an epidemic, then to identify methods of determining those at highest risk, then to dissect the toxicity of individual agents, and finally to monitor the effects of introducing newer and safer therapies. The response of industry, academia, the Food and Drug Administration, and others to this problem has been in many ways exemplary, and should be rewarded by substantial improvements in public health.

REFERENCES

1. Fries JF, Williams CA, Bloch DA, Michel BA. Nonsteroidal anti-inflammatory drug associated gastropathy: Incidence and risk factor models. *Am J Med*. 1991;91:213–22.
2. Fries JF, Spitz PW, Kraines RG, Holman HR. Measurement of patient outcome in arthritis. *Arthritis Rheum*. 1980;23:137–45.
3. Fries JF. The ARAMIS (American Rheumatism Association Medical Information System) post-marketing surveillance program. *Drug Info J*. 1985;19:257–62.
4. Fries FJ, Spitz PW, Williams CA, Bloch DA, Singh G, Hubert HB. A toxicity index for comparison of side effects among different drugs. *Arthritis Rheum*. 1990;33,121–30.
5. Singh G, Ramey DR. NSAID-induced gastrointestinal complications: The ARAMIS perspective – 1997. *J Rheum*. 1998;25(suppl 51):8–16.
6. Singh G, Ramey DR, Morfeld D, Shi H, Hatoum H, Fries JF. Gastrointestinal tract complications of non-steroidal anti-inflammatory drug treatment in rheumatoid arthritis. A prospective observational cohort study. *Arch Intern Med*. 1996;156:1530–6.
7. Fries JF. NSAID gastropathy: the second most deadly rheumatic disease? Epidemiology and risk appraisal. *J Rheumatol*. 1991;18(suppl 28):6–10.
8. Avorn J, Solomon D, Levin R, Lo J. Epidemiologic analysis of prophylactic drug use and NSAID gastropathy. *Arthritis Rheum*. 1996;39(suppl):S165.
9. Fries JF, Ramey DR, Singh G, Morfeld D, Bloch DA, Raynauld JP et al. A reevaluation of aspirin therapy in rheumatoid arthritis (RA). *Arch Intern Med*. 1993;153:2465–71.

10. Henry DH, Lim LL-Y, Garcia Rodriguez L, Gutthann SP, Carson JL, Griffin M. Variability in risk of gastrointestinal complications with individual non-steroidal anti-inflammatory drugs: results of a collaborative meta-analysis. *Br Med J*. 1996;312:1563–6.

11. Distel M, Mueller C, Bluhmki E, Fries JF. Safety of meloxicam: A global analysis of clinical trials. *Br J Rheumatol*. 1996;35(suppl 1):68–77.

12. Fries JF. Reevaluating the therapeutic approach to rheumatoid arthritis: the "sawtooth" strategy. *J Rheumatol*. 1990;17(suppl 22):12–15.

13. Fries JF. The toxicity of anti-rheumatic drugs: Problems and solutions. *Proc R Coll Physicians Edinb*. 1995;25:398–405.

7

Experimental basis for non-steroidal anti-inflammatory drug-induced gut injury

B. J. R. WHITTLE

Ever since the introduction of salicylates into medicine at the beginning of the 20th century, their side effects on the stomach and intestine have been documented, although much of the early evidence was somewhat anecdotal. Over the past decade convincing evidence has accumulated from epidemiological studies and direct clinical trials to confirm that chronic use of aspirin and other non-steroidal anti-inflammatory drugs (NSAIDs) gives rise to serious toxic actions in the gastrointestinal tract, including haemorrhage and ulcers, in a large proportion of the patient population, particularly the elderly. These recent advances in clinical knowledge and recognition of the substantial problems associated with such compounds have been accompanied by a significant change in our understanding of the basic mechanisms underlying these damaging actions.

Several methods for determining gastrointestinal damage and bleeding have been used in the clinical evaluation of such compounds, including the measurement of faecal output of radiotagged erythrocytes, measurement of back-diffusion or acid loss, and the evaluation of ion flux across the mucosa with accompanying changes in transepithelial potential difference (PD). It is clear, however, that direct visual inspection by endoscopy is of major importance in determining the toxic effects of NSAIDs on the gastric and duodenal mucosa.

Over 60 years ago, a gastroscopic study on the effect of aspirin on the human stomach showed the deleterious properties of this compound on the gastric mucosa[1]. During the past decade, the direct gastric effects of many of the clinically used anti-inflammatory agents, including aspirin, naproxen and indomethacin, have been investigated by endoscopic techniques. All of these compounds caused visible gastric mucosal damage and erosion formation to various degrees, depending on the dosage regimen. However, experiences from experimental studies have indicated that simple macroscopic observation may not reveal mucosal defects that would be apparent on histological examination of biopsy samples. Thus, some caution must be applied to the interpretation of all such macroscopic data, especially regarding claims for the absence of any toxic effects on the stomach of novel agents. It is likely, however, that any minor defects, such as epithelial disruption, may readily be repaired over a short time, although repair processes, such as restitution of the epithelial layer, may also be affected by these agents.

TOPICAL IRRITATION AND GASTRIC MUCOSAL DAMAGE

An important concept concerning the effects of topically applied salicylates on the gastric mucosa was developed by Davenport and colleagues in the mid-1960s[2], and has been largely upheld over the past 30 years. The ability of topically administered aspirin and related salicylates to promote acid back-diffusion into the canine gastric mucosa was clearly demonstrated in early experiments[3] and has been amply confirmed by many workers using different species and models, both in vivo and in vitro. The increase in acid loss is accompanied by an increase in luminal sodium ion concentration, and the efflux of potassium ions into the gastric human lumen and the transmucosal flux of non-ionic moieties can also be enhanced by topical irritants (Figure 1).

The transmural PD across the gastric mucosa has been used as an index of the integrity of the gastric mucosa in animals and man. A reduction in gastric PD has been observed after the topical application of irritants such as aspirin in man. This occurs concurrently with the other characteristics of gastric 'barrier' damage, such as the back-diffusion of acid from the gastric lumen into the mucosa, which correlate with histologically demonstrable damage to the human mucosa after

Figure 1 Acid back-diffusion and ion flux across the gastric mucosa following topical irritation by NSAIDs

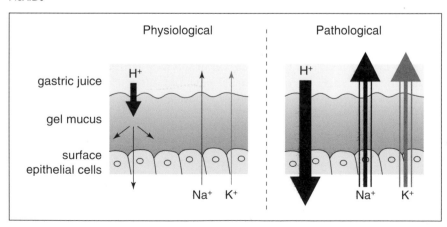

aspirin ingestion[4]. It is likely that changes in PD reflect damage to the superficial epithelial cells, while restoration of PD accompanies the process of rapid restitution of the damaged epithelium following local injury[5].

The barrier changes following aspirin or salicylate application to the mucosa extend not only to other NSAIDs such as indomethacin, but also to other local irritants such as bile acids and salts or ethanol. The action of these agents, not generally regarded as cyclooxygenase (COX) inhibitors, suggests that this barrier-breaking activity is not directly related to the inhibition of prostaglandin biosynthesis. Furthermore, intravenous administration of aspirin to animals or humans failed to elicit barrier damage[6], as determined by luminal acid loss or PD measurements, indicating that such changes are the result of local contact with the mucosal tissue and not a reflection of COX inhibition.

Since early studies indicated that such barrier-breaking activities of aspirin and salicylate occurred under acid conditions in the stomach, it has been suggested that absorption of the unionized form of these carboxylic acids is involved in the damage, although the presence of hydrogen ions in the gastric lumen appears very important. It was proposed from early studies that salicylate anions could be trapped in the mucosal cells during absorption, but their contribution to mucosal injury is not known.

It has been proposed that acidification of the mucosal interstitial tissue following challenge with NSAIDs leads to the observed cellular damage. Subsequent studies indicated that the barrier-breaking activity of these drugs resulted from epithelial disruption, perhaps as a consequence of local metabolic actions, including uncoupling of oxidative phosphorylation in the epithelium[7].

Approaches to reducing the direct topical gastric damage of the NSAIDs have involved modification of the free carboxyl substituents, which have been implicated as a factor in these toxic actions. Esterification of this moiety, as in methyl aspirin, has provided compounds with less ulcerogenic action following intragastric administration, while anti-inflammatory activity is retained, presumably following liberation of the free acid by the action of plasma esterases[7]. While such modifications may reduce direct local irritancy, these chemically modified compounds, once activated in the systemic circulation, for example by de-esterification, could retain their biochemical actions, including actions on gastric COX, which may lead to more chronic development of gastrointestinal disturbances. This chemical masking of the free carboxylic acid grouping may also contribute to the gastric-sparing actions of the recently described nitric oxide (NO)-containing NSAIDs[8].

LUMINAL SURFACE LAYERS

The mucus layer offers little buffering capacity and appears readily permeable to acid. However, it can act as a lubricant and barrier to physical damage such as that induced by local tissue contact with fragments of anti-inflammatory tablets.

This layer can also impede the back-diffusion of hydrogen ions, creating an unstirred layer of water and electrolytes, notably bicarbonate, at the apical membrane[9]. It has been suggested that NSAIDs may affect mucus biosynthesis, as well as alkaline secretion, and could therefore contribute to the process of ulceration by attenuating the elaboration of this local more alkaline environment, making the underlying tissue more susceptible to damage.

It has also been proposed that the mucosa is protected from attack by luminal acid by the water-repellent properties of the luminal surface. This hydrophobicity of the mucosal surface, previously attributed to a layer of surface-active phospholipids, has now been shown to be largely dependent on surface mucus gel[10]. This hydrophobicity was substantially reduced by topical application of aspirin, which may reflect the inhibition of mucus and bicarbonate secretion[10]. Such changes could thus augment acid back-diffusion and contribute to the local irritant actions of aspirin and other NSAIDs.

Despite all this information on the luminal actions of these agents, it is clear that NSAIDs can provoke gastro–duodenal toxicity by mechanisms other than topical actions, since many of these agents cause extensive lesions following parenteral administration. It has been proposed that the mechanism of such systemic actions involves the inhibition of COX[11] reducing the production of protective prostanoids such as prostaglandin E_2 (PGE_2) and prostacyclin (see reference 12).

COX-1 INHIBITION AND GASTRIC INJURY

Role of COX-1 Products

Endogenous metabolites of arachidonic acid, formed via COX-1 have been implicated as local mediators or modulators of gastric mucosal function. Prostaglandins of the E and I series, PGE_2 and prostacyclin respectively, are formed by gastric mucosal tissue. These prostanoids can inhibit gastric acid secretion, stimulate gastric bicarbonate and mucus secretion, induce vasodilatation in the mucosal microcirculation, prevent the vascular stasis induced by damaging agents, and affect sodium and chloride ionic flux. These prostanoids and their synthetic analogues protect the gastric mucosa from damage, an action which may be brought about by their effect on several of the above parameters[13–16].

Since prostanoids exert such potent actions on gastric function and integrity, particularly from COX-1 inhibition, it is not surprising that alterations in local prostaglandin formation have been implicated as a mechanism underlying gastric damage and disease. The depletion of endogenous prostanoids by NSAIDs is a likely mechanism contributing to the gastric mucosal damage induced by these drugs, both in experimental models and in clinical use.

Effects of NSAIDs on Mucosal Prostanoid Production

Early studies demonstrated that indomethacin at ulcerogenic doses reduced the level of prostaglandins in homogenates of rat gastric mucosa. When administered in divided doses over 24 hours, a range of clinically used NSAIDs, including indomethacin, flurbiprofen and naproxen, induced a comparable degree of gastric erosion formation, which paralleled the inhibition of mucosal prostacyclin production[17]. In contrast, sodium salicylate or an experimental agent did not inhibit mucosal COX or cause macroscopic damage, further supporting the association between these two events (Figure 2).

Site-selective Inhibition of Prostanoid Formation: COX-1 and COX-2

In early studies on the possible differential inhibition of COX, it was demonstrated that prostanoid production in inflammatory sites could be inhibited without affecting prostanoid generation in the gastric mucosa (Figure 2). Moreover, such selective inhibition in the inflammatory areas by certain anti-inflammatory agents did not provoke gastric mucosal injury[17]. These studies led to the proposal that there may be different isoforms of COX at the inflammatory sites and in the gastric mucosa that would be susceptible to pharmacological exploitation. The contribution of any pharmacokinetic disposition to the site-selectivity of the agents studied was not known, nor whether it reflected uptake or selectivity of action of the agents on the inflammatory cells. However, the findings did indicate the potential for site-selective COX inhibitors to yield anti-inflammatory agents with less gastrointestinal toxicity[17].

*Figure 2 Gastric mucosal damage and the inhibition of COX products in the rat gastric mucosa and inflammatory exudate induced by NSAIDs. Drugs were administered orally three times over 24 hours, and prostacyclin formation in gastric mucosal strips ex vivo and PGE$_2$ levels in carrageenan-induced inflammatory exudate in an implanted sponge were determined. Gastric mucosal damage was assessed macroscopically and expressed as an index of damage. Results are shown as mean±S.E.M. of 5–12 experiments. A significant difference from control (P<0.01) is shown as *. Data are adapted from Whittle et al.[17].*

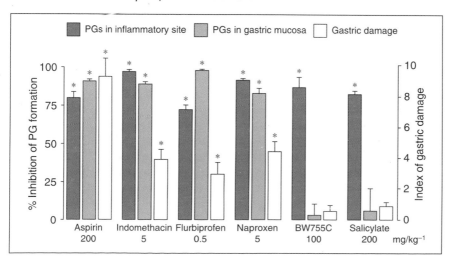

The identification some 10 years later, using molecular and biochemical technology, of the two isoforms of COX[18–20], has provided a rational approach for the development of selective COX inhibitors. The isoform referred to as COX-1 has been identified as a constitutive enzyme, inhibition of which leads to gastrointestinal mucosal injury. Production of prostanoids at the site of inflammation is now attributed predominantly to the expression of an inducible enzyme, COX-2. Selective inhibition of COX-2, while not impairing the physiological production of protective prostanoids by the COX-1 enzyme, has provided a new pharmacological approach to the identification of safer anti-inflammatory drugs.

Interaction of COX-1 Inhibition With Local Irritancy

Experimental studies have demonstrated that topical irritant actions and COX-1 inhibition can synergistically interact to provoke more extensive mucosal injury than that by either process alone (Figure 3). Thus inhibition of COX-1 greatly augments the injury provoked by locally acting irritants, which may involve actions on the gastro–duodenal microcirculation[12]. It has also been proposed that adherence of neutrophils to the microvasculature is involved in the early events leading to gastric mucosal damage, a process that could involve inhibition of COX-1[8,21]. The potency of anti-inflammatory agents for inducing gastric lesions could therefore depend both on their activity as barrier breakers and as COX inhibitors, with both actions independently having the potential to lead to gastric damage, but interacting synergistically to provoke more extensive ulceration.

EFFECTS ON THE INTESTINE

Although the actions of aspirin and related compounds on the gastric or duodenal mucosa have been the more extensively studied and reported, such

Figure 3 Interactive mechanisms in the pathogenesis of gastric mucosal damage induced by COX-1 inhibitors

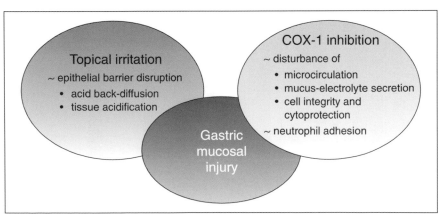

agents are also well known to cause or promote damage in the small and large intestine. In rats, indomethacin induces the development of chronic lesions in the jejunum and ileum after 1–3 days of acute or chronic administration, leading to extensive inflammation and eventual intestinal perforation and death[22,23]. Bacterial invasion from the lumen appears to be involved in the eventual process of tissue damage[22], which may be aided by reduction in prostanoid biosynthesis.

Acute administration of aspirin suspension to humans rapidly produces erythrocyte extrusion and focal erosion of the jejunal villi determined by electron microscopy[24]. Chronic ingestion of NSAIDs has also been associated with damage to the small intestinal mucosa. Thus, oral ingestion of aspirin, ibuprofen or indomethacin by healthy volunteers increased the permeability of the small intestine to radiolabelled markers[25,26]. This effect was also observed after rectal administration of these agents, indicating that this was a systemic action and not just a reflection of any local irritant effect. Moreover, in studies on patients receiving NSAIDs for the treatment of rheumatoid arthritis or osteoarthritis, over 60% exhibited blood and protein loss with demonstrable inflammation of the small intestine[25,26]. The degree of mucosal inflammation was milder than that observed in patients with Crohn's ileitis, although the radiologically detected abnormalities in the ileum suggest that ulceration and strictures could ultimately develop on chronic administration of these agents[25,26].

It has been proposed that inhibition of COX-1, along with local irritant actions, contributes to the process of cellular injury in the intestinal mucosa. However, the potential involvement of bacterial products had not been fully explained. It is known that lipopolysaccharide (LPS) derived from bacterial endotoxin can induce the formation of cytotoxic or pro-inflammatory mediators. The cytotoxic actions of NO formed by the inducible isoform of NO synthase (iNOS), which is expressed following exposure to LPS of a range of gut cell types including inflammatory and epithelial cells, have been described[27].

The role of iNOS in the chronic generation of intestinal injury and inflammation provoked by NSAIDs has recently been investigated[28]. Indomethacin, flurbiprofen or naproxen provoked a substantial elevation of vascular leakage of plasma and lesion formation in the rat jejunum over 48 hours, commencing 18 hours after administration, associated with the induction of iNOS. Administration of the broad spectrum antibiotic ampicillin inhibited both the expression of iNOS and the plasma leakage observed over 48 hours after the NSAIDs. Likewise, administration of polymyxin-B, which binds and inactivates LPS, also prevented iNOS expression and intestinal injury. These findings thus suggest that expression of iNOS following administration of these NSAIDs involves the liberation of LPS from gut bacteria and leads to the chronic development of microvascular injury and tissue damage to the small intestine[28]. The early events that give rise to the breach in the mucosal defence mechanisms, allowing the ingress of gut bacteria, appear to involve the inhibition of COX-1, and could reflect local microcirculatory actions and epithelial dysfunction.

CONCLUSIONS

It is apparent, therefore, that the mechanisms underlying the gastrointestinal injury by NSAIDs are complex and distinct, being specific to different regions of the gut. However, the mechanisms of injury appear to involve the inhibition of COX-1, although other processes may play interactive roles in the pathogenesis of the tissue damage. Advances in our understanding of these processes have allowed the development of novel agents, the COX-2-selective inhibitory agents, that should have more beneficial anti-inflammatory actions with reduced propensity for gut toxicity.

REFERENCES

1. Douthwaite AH, Lintott GM. Gastroscopic observation of the effects of aspirin and certain other substances on the stomach. *Lancet.* 1935;2:1222–5.
2. Davenport HW. Gastric mucosal injury by fatty and acetylsalicylic acids. *Gastroenterology.* 1964;46:245–53.
3. Davenport HW. Fluid protection by the gastric mucosa during damage by acetic and salicylic acids. *Gastroenterology.* 1966;50:487–99.
4. Bowen BK, Krause WJ, Ivey KJ. Effect of sodium bicarbonate on aspirin-induced damage and potential difference changes in human gastric mucosa. *Br Med J.* 1977;2:1052–4.
5. Wallace JL, Whittle BJR. Role of mucus in the repair of gastric epithelial cell damage in the rat. *Gastroenterology.* 1986;91:603–11.
6. Grossman MI, Matsumota KK, Lichter RJ. Fecal blood loss by oral and intravenous administration of various salicylates. *Gastroenterology.* 1961;40:383–8.
7. Rainsford KD, Whitehouse MW. Anti-inflammatory anti-pyretic salicylic acid esters, with low gastric ulcerogenic activity. *Agents Actions.* 1980;10:451–6.
8. Wallace JL. Non-steroidal anti-inflammatory drugs and gastroenteropathy: The second hundred years. *Gastroenterology.* 1997;112:1000–16.
9. Allen A, Garner A. Mucus and bicarbonate secretion in the stomach and their possible role in mucosal protection. *Gut.* 1980;21:249–62.
10. Goddard PJ, Kao YJ, Lightenberger LM. Luminal surface hydrophobicity of canine gastric mucosa is dependent on a surface mucous gel. *Gastroenterology.* 1990;98:361–70.
11. Vane JR. Inhibition of prostaglandin synthesis as a mechanism of action for aspirin-like drugs. *Nat New Biol.* 1971;231:232–5.
12. Whittle BJR. Unwanted effects of aspirin and related agents in the gastrointestinal tract. In: Vane JR, Botting RM, editors. *Aspirin and Other Salicylates.* London: Chapman and Hall; 1992;465–509.
13. Robert A, Nezamis JE, Lancaster C, Hanchar AJ. Cytoprotection by prostaglandins in rats – prevention of gastric necrosis produced by alcohol, HCl, NaOH, hypertonic NaCl and thermal injury. *Gastroenterology.* 1979;77:433–43.
14. Main IHM, Whittle BJR. Investigation of the vasodilator and antisecretory role of prostaglandins in the rat gastric mucosa by use of non-steroidal anti-inflammatory drugs. *Br J Pharmacol.* 1975;53:217–24.
15. Whittle BJR. Mechanisms underlying gastric mucosal damage induced by indomethacin and bile salt, and the actions of prostaglandins. *Br J Pharmacol.* 1997;60:455–60.
16. Whittle BJR, Vane JR. Prostanoids as regulators of gastrointestinal function. In: Johnson LR editor. *Physiology of the Gastrointestinal Tract (Second Edition).* New York: Raven Press; 1987;143–80.

17. Whittle BJR, Higgs GA, Eakins KE, Moncada S, Vane JR. Selective inhibition of prostaglandin production in inflammatory exudates and gastric mucosa. *Nature.* 1980;284:271–3.
18. Fu J-Y, Masferrer JL, Seibert K, Raz A, Needleman P. The induction and suppression of prostaglandin H_2 synthase (cyclooxygenase) in human monocytes. *J Biol Chem.* 1990;265:16737–40.
19. Xie W, Chipman JG, Robertson DL, Erikson RL, Simmons DL. Expression of a mitogen-responsive gene encoding prostaglandin synthase is regulated by mRNA splicing. *Proc Natl Acad Sci USA.* 1991;88:2692–6.
20. O'Banion MK, Sadowski HB, Winn V, Young DA. A serum- and glucocorticoid-regulated 4-kilobase mRNA encodes a cyclooxygenase-related protein. *J Biol Chem.* 1991;266:23261–7.
21. Wallace JL, Keenan CM, Granger DN. Gastric ulceration induced by non-steroidal anti-inflammatory drugs is a neutrophil-dependent process. *Am J Physiol.* 1990;259:G462–G467.
22. Robert A. An intestinal disease produced experimentally by a prostaglandin deficiency. *Gastroenterology.* 1975;69:1045–7.
23. Whittle BJR. Temporal relationship between cyclo-oxygenase inhibition, as measured by prostacyclin biosynthesis, and the gastrointestinal damage induced by indomethacin in the rat. *Gastroenterology.* 1981;80:94–8.
24. Ivey KJ, Baskin WN, Krause WJ, Terry B. Effect of aspirin and acid on human jejunal mucosa. An ultrastructural study. *Gastroenterology.* 1979;76:50–6.
25. Bjarnason I, Prouse P, Smith T, Gumpel MJ, Zanelli G, Smethurst P et al. Blood and protein loss via small-intestinal inflammation induced by non-steroidal anti-inflammatory drugs. *Lancet.* 1987;ii:711–4.
26. Bjarnason I, Zanelli G, Smith T, Prouse P, Williams P, Smethurst P et al. Non-steroidal anti-inflammatory drug-induced intestinal inflammation in humans. *Gastroenterology.* 1987;93:480–9.
27. Whittle BJR. Nitric oxide – a mediator of inflammation and mucosal defence. *Eur J Gastroenterol Hepatol.* 1997;9:1026–32.
28. Whittle BJR, Laszlo F, Evans SM, Moncada S. Induction of nitric oxide synthase and microvascular injury in the rat jejunum provoked by indomethacin. *Br J Pharmacol.* 1995;116:2286–90.

8

Gastrointestinal effects of non-steroidal anti-inflammatory drugs

C. J. HAWKEY

Widespread synthesis of aspirin dates from a description published by Felix Hoffman in 1897[1]. He was stimulated to try to devise a better tolerated form of salicylic acid because his father had indigestion when he took salicylic acid. This may not be surprising given that this compound is now used for destruction of warts. Although Hoffman's acetylation of salicylic acid made the compound better tolerated symptomatically, by 1937 it was clear that it was toxic to the gastric mucosa, causing acute erosions and chronic ulcers[2]. Attempts in the 1960s and 70s to produce better tolerated forms of aspirin in the shape of the non-aspirin non-steroidal anti-inflammatory drugs (NSAIDs) also proved unsuccessful, and these drugs are now recognized as a major cause of gastrotoxicity[3,4].

EFFECTS OF ASPIRIN AND NSAIDS ON THE STOMACH AND DUODENUM

Acute Injury
Acute injury, coming on within 90 minutes of ingestion, is almost universal with aspirin, and even with 75 mg aspirin about one-third of subjects will have acute erosions and petechiae[5]. Acute injury with non-aspirin NSAIDs is less florid and comes on somewhat more slowly[6].

Chronic Ingestion – Endoscopic Studies
Nevertheless, endoscopic studies have shown about one-fifth of patients taking non-aspirin NSAIDs to have a peptic ulcer, usually silent and with a 2:1 predominance for gastric over duodenal. It seems that ulcer development and its site

of expression may be influenced by a number of factors including the patient's sex and *Helicobacter pylori* status. In a recently presented analysis of lesions found at baseline in two large clinical trials, patients infected with *H. pylori*, those with a past history and those over the age of 60 were more likely to present with ulcers than erosions. *H. pylori* was associated with duodenal as opposed to gastric ulcers and this was also associated with male sex, independent of *H. pylori* status[7]. However, 44% of all duodenal ulcers were in patients who were *H. pylori* negative, establishing finally that NSAIDs do indeed cause duodenal ulceration rather than provoking relapse of ulcers associated with *H. pylori* infection.

By following patients who continued to take NSAIDs during ulcer healing and up to 6 months thereafter, we found that the site and nature (ulcer or multiple erosions) of the initial lesion were highly likely to be replicated at relapse[8,9]. More than two-thirds of all relapses were with the same lesion and at the same site as had initially presented. General risk factors such as *H. pylori* status did not increase the risk of relapse. The site-specific nature of relapse therefore suggests that past history is mediated via a mucosal defect rather than a general risk factor such as *H. pylori* infection and explains the paradox that NSAID ulcers are more common in patients with a past history, whilst ulcers (particularly gastric ulcers) are as common in those who are *H. pylori* positive as in those who are *H. pylori* negative[10].

Ulcer Complications

NSAID ulcers are important principally because they predispose to ulcer complications. Approximately 4000 deaths per annum in the United Kingdom are attributed to peptic ulcer. Several studies suggest that 30% of ulcer complications are attributed to the use of NSAIDs, suggesting that these drugs may cause the death of 1200 patients per annum in the United Kingdom[3]. Risk factors that are well recognized as predisposing to ulcer complications are old age, past history, high NSAID dose, and simultaneous use of warfarin or steroids. It is now also clear that some NSAIDs such as azapropazone, piroxicam or ketoprofen are associated with higher rates of ulcer complications than others such as ibuprofen[11]. Whether this relates entirely to effective dose is not known but it is clear that seemingly less toxic NSAIDs can become more toxic if used in higher doses.

We have recently completed and published in abstract form a study evaluating further the relative role of *H. pylori* and NSAIDs in the development of ulcer bleeding in Nottingham[12]. In this study patients were matched to controls admitted to hospital for reasons that would not be influenced by NSAID use. *H. pylori* status, and whether the organism was virulent (as indexed by being positive for cytotoxin associated gene, or *cagA*) were established serologically and NSAID use by prospective structured interview. Only *cagA*-positive *H. pylori* were associated with ulcer bleeding. NSAID use was strongly associated with both gastric and duodenal ulceration. In contrast to previous studies, aspirin use accounted for more ulcer bleeds than all other NSAIDs put together and nearly all of this was attributed to use of aspirin in doses of 300 mg per day or less. Both gastric (particularly) and duodenal ulcer were increased by NSAID use.

Type C Gastritis

Some 40% of NSAID users have a curious hyperplastic histological change in the antrum characterized by foveolar hyperplasia, capillary congestion, oedema and smooth muscle hyperplasia[4]. Type C gastritis is itself asymptomatic and it is controversial whether it predisposes to subsequent ulceration. Its cause is uncertain but a similar pattern is seen in patients with bile reflux and it is believed that type C gastritis in NSAID users represents an exacerbation of this process by reflux of NSAIDs from the duodenum to the stomach, possibly associated with enterohepatic re-circulation.

LESIONS IN THE LARGE AND SMALL BOWEL

Ileal Valves

A rare but apparently specific association with NSAID use is the development of valve-like lesions in the ileum. Histologically these are somewhat like type C gastritis with smooth muscle hyperplasia. They are associated with obstruction and a high mortality, but are very rare[13].

Small Bowel Ulceration

More common is small bowel ulceration. In rats given a high enough dose of indomethacin, deep necrotic ulceration with secondary infection is the usual cause of death. Small bowel ulceration is much less common in humans, but enteroscopy and post-mortem studies have suggested a prevalence of about 10% in NSAID users[14,15]. The extent to which these (in humans often superficial) ulcers contribute to pathology is not fully defined but chronic anaemia and hypoproteinaemia have been attributed to small bowel damage[16] and several case reports associate use of certain NSAIDs including diclofenac with deep ulceration in the ileo–caecal region[17]. Epidemiological studies also suggest that NSAID use is associated with a 2–3-fold increase in small bowel perforation[18,19].

NSAIDs and Ulcerative Colitis

Use of analgesics (including NSAIDs, but also paracetamol) was associated with colitis many years ago[20]. It has remained controversial whether this is causal or consequential (with patients taking NSAIDs in response to the early symptoms of relapse). Two recent studies, including one involving patients presenting with colitis for the first time raised the possibility that the relationship is indeed causal[21–23].

POSSIBLE INDUCTION OF CYCLOOXYGENASE (COX)-2 IN THE HUMAN GASTROINTESTINAL TRACT

Ulcerative Colitis

Early studies suggested that active ulcerative colitis was associated with increased levels of a steroid-suppressible form of COX[24]. Induction of COX-2 in ulcerative colitis has been confirmed by the demonstration of COX-2 mRNA in relapse of ulcerative colitis using reverse transcriptase-polymerase chain reaction (RT-PCR)[25]. These observations may have implications for the use of selective COX-2 inhibitors. Given at the time of relapse when COX-2 is induced, they have the potential to worsen colitis as with non-selective NSAIDs. However, they may have advantages over non-selective NSAIDs if prostaglandin synthesis during remission is of critical importance for prevention of relapse, since they should not inhibit prostaglandin synthesis under these circumstances.

H. pylori

Induction of COX-2 in inflammatory bowel disease raises the possibility that COX-2 may be induced in the human gastrointestinal tract under other circumstances. In particular, *H. pylori* has been shown to be associated with increased prostaglandin synthesis[26]. However, as yet, it has not been possible to show clearly that this activity is prevented by COX-2 rather than COX-1 inhibitors[27].

Ulcer Rim

Animal studies have shown that acute induction of erosions by aspirin and chronic ulceration caused by acetic acid are both associated with induction of COX-2[28], whilst both non-selective NSAIDs and selective COX-2 inhibitors (albeit at high dose) impair healing of cryo ulcers and reduce popularity of their granulation tissue[29]. This reflects human data showing reduced vascularity of NSAID-associated ulcers compared with *H. pylori* ulcers[30]. Ongoing work from our Department has shown histological evidence of COX-2 induction in macrophages, fibroblasts and endothelial cells in granulation tissue[31]. We have also isolated human gastric endothelial cells and shown by immunofluorescence, Western blotting and RT-PCR that these cells are capable of expressing both COX-1 and COX-2, and that COX-2 expression is enhanced when such cells form microvascular circles under the influence of matrigel or phorbol ester[32]. Similarly, myofibroblasts and macrophages harvested from partially disaggregated gastric mucosal biopsy samples have been shown to be capable of synthesizing large quantities of prostaglandins and expressing COX-1 and COX-2[33].

Gastrointestinal Cancer

Several epidemiological studies suggest that the benefits of aspirin and non-aspirin NSAIDs in protecting against gastrointestinal cancer are not restricted to the colon but are also seen for gastric cancer[34–36]. The mechanisms by which COX-2 is associated with the development of malignancy in stomach and duodenum and how this observation relates to the therapeutic benefits of aspirin and non-aspirin NSAIDs are far from clear.

However, two observations are important. When stimulated by transforming growth factor-α, the human colonocyte cell line HCA7, clone 29, increases its expression of COX-2 and makes substantial quantities of prostaglandin E_2[37]. As in other cell lines this enhancement is particularly evident in the perinuclear area, and confocal microscopy suggests that activity may also be present within the nucleus[37]. This proximity of COX-2 to the nucleus raises the possibility that products of COX-2 may exert their effects in an intracrine way, for example by binding to the peroxisome proliferator-activated nuclear receptors[38]. Alternatively, some actions may be exerted in an autocrine way via released prostaglandins. A third possibility is a paracrine action. In this context, it should be noted that in some malignant tumours increased levels of COX-2 in the stroma rather than the malignant epithelium have been reported[39]. A final paradox that may need to be resolved before the role of COX-2 in cancer is fully understood relates to the fact that aspirin, a drug which more effectively inhibits COX-1 than COX-2, is beneficial in colonic and gastric cancer.

SUMMARY AND CONCLUSIONS

Aspirin and non-aspirin NSAIDs have toxic effects throughout the gastrointestinal tract. The greatest number of problems arise from their ability to ulcerate the stomach and duodenum. Selective COX-2 inhibitors are likely to reduce this toxicity but there may be some limitations. In particular it is possible that they may be ulcerogenic in some patients with *H. pylori* infection. They may retard the healing of existing ulcers and they may be harmful at some phases of inflammatory bowel disease. Conversely, induction of COX-2 in gastric and colonic tumours suggests a therapeutic role for these drugs in this context.

REFERENCES

1. Mann CC, Plummer ML. *The Aspirin Wars, Money, Medicine and 100 Years of Rampant Competition*. Boston: Harvard Business School Press; 1991.
2. Douthwaite A, Lintott CA. Gastroscopic observations of the effect of aspirin and certain other substances on the stomach. *Lancet*. 1938;2:1222.
3. Hawkey CJ. Non-steroidal anti-inflammatory drugs and ulcers: Facts and figures multiply, but do they add up? *Br Med J*. 1990;300:278–84.
4. Hawkey CJ, Hudson N. Mucosal injury caused by drugs, chemicals and stress. In: *Bockus Gastroenterology 5th Edition*. Haubrich WS, Schaffner F, Berk JE, editors. Philadelphia: WB Saunders Co.; 1994;656–99.
5. Hawkey CJ, Hawthorne AB, Hudson N, Cole AT, Mahida YR, Daneshmend TK. Separation of aspirin's impairment of haemostasis from mucosal injury in the human stomach. *Clin Sci*. 1991;81:565–73.
6. Hawkey CJ, O'Morain C, Murray FE, McCarthy C, Tiernay D, Devane J. Two comparative endoscopic evaluations of naprelan. *Am J Orthop*. 1996;25(9S):30–6.
7. Hawkey CJ, Swannell AJ, Naesdal J, Walan A, Yeomans ND. Influence of sex and *Helicobacter pylori* on type and location of lesions in NSAID users. *Gastroenterology*. 1998;114:A145;G0595.
8. Hawkey CJ, Jeffrey AK, Szczepanski L, Walker DG, Barkun A, Swannell AJ et al. for the OMNIUM Study Group. A comparison of omeprazole and misoprostol for treating and preventing ulcers associated with non-steroidal anti-inflammatory drugs. *N Engl J Med*. 1998;338:727–34.

9. Yeomans ND, Tulassay Z, Juhasz L, Racz I, Howard JM, van Rensburg CJ et al. for the ASTRONAUT Study Group. A comparison of omeprazole and ranitidine for treating and preventing ulcers associated with non-steroidal anti-inflammatory drugs. *N Engl J Med*. 1998;338:719–26.

10. Cullen DJE, Hawkey GM, Greenwood DC, Humphreys H, Shepherd V, Logan RFA et al. Peptic ulcer bleeding: relative roles of *Helicobacter pylori* and non-steroidal anti-inflammatory drugs. *Gut*. 1997;41:459–62.

11. Henry D, Lim LL-Y, García Rodríguez LA, Gutthann SP, Carson JL, Griffin M et al. Variability in risk of gastrointestinal complications with individual non steroidal anti-inflammatory drugs: results of a collaborative meta-analysis. *Br Med J*. 1996;312:1563–6.

12. Hawkey GM, Stack WA, Cole AT, Long RG, Logan RFA, Hawkey CJ. Blood in the stomach as a surrogate for clinical end points in GI bleeding trials. *Gastroenterology*. 1998;114:A146:G0598.

13. Bjarnason I, Price AB, Zanelli G. Clinicopathological features of non steroidal anti-inflammatory drug induced small intestinal strictures. *Gastroenterology*. 1998;94:1074–4.

14. Allison MC, Howatson AG, Torrance CJ, Lee FD, Russell RI. Gastrointestinal damage associated with the use of non steroidal anti-inflammatory drugs. *N Engl J Med*. 1992;327:749–54.

15. Morris AJ, Madhok R, Sturrock RD, Capell HA, MacKenzie JF. Enteroscopic diagnosis of small bowel ulceration in patients receiving non steroidal anti-inflammatory drugs. *Lancet*. 1991;337:520.

16. Bjarnason I, Zanelli G, Prouse P, Smethurst P, Smith T, Levi S et al. Blood and protein loss via small intestinal inflammation induced by non steroidal anti-inflammatory drugs. *Lancet*. 1987;ii:711–4.

17. Hudson N, Wilkinson MJ, Swannell AJ, Steele RJ, Hawkey CJ. Ileo–caecal ulceration associated with the use of diclofenac retard. *Aliment Pharmacol Ther*. 1993;7:197–200.

18. Langman MJS, Morgan L, Worral A. Use of anti-inflammatory drugs by patients admitted with small or large bowel perforation and haemorrhage. *Br Med J*. 1985;290:347–9.

19. Campbell K, Steele RJC. Non steroidal anti-inflammatory drugs and complicated diverticular disease: A case control study. *Br J Surg*. 1991;78:190–1.

20. Rampton DS, McNeil NI, Sarner M. Analgesic ingestion and other factors preceding relapse in ulcerative colitis. *Gut*. 1983;24:187–9.

21. Gibson GR. Colitis induced by non steroidal anti-inflammatory drugs. *Arch Intern Med*. 1992;152:625–32.

22. Evans JMM, McMahon AD, Murray FE, McDevitt DG, MacDonald TM. Non steroidal anti-inflammatory drugs are associated with emergency admission to hospital for colitis due to inflammatory bowel disease. *Gut*. 1997;40:619–22.

23. Gleeson MH, Hardman JV, Clinton C. Colitis, non steroidal anti-inflammatory drugs (NSAIDs) and salicylates – a strong association. *Gut*. 1996;39(suppl 3):A243, Abstract 1479.

24. Hawkey CJ. Evidence that prednisolone is inhibitory to the cyclooxygenase activity of human rectal mucosa. *Prostaglandins*. 1982;23:397–410.

25. McLaughlan J, Seth R, Cole AT, Scott BB, Jenkins D, Robins AR et al. Increased inducible cyclooxygenase associated with treatment failure in ulcerative colitis. *Gut*. 1996;38:A58.

26. Hudson N, Balsitis M, Filipowicz B, Hawkey CJ. Effect of *Helicobacter pylori* colonisation on gastric mucosal eicosanoid synthesis in patients taking non-steroidal anti-inflammatory drugs. *Gut*. 1993;34:748–51.

27. Jackson LM, Wu K, Mahida YR, Jenkins D, Donnelly MT, Hawkey CJ. COX-1 expression in human gastric mucosa infected with *Helicobacter pylori*: constitutive or induced? *Gastroenterology*. 1998;114:A160:G0653.

28. Mizuno H, Sakamoto C, Matsuda K, Wada K, Uchida T, Noguchi H et al. Induction of cyclooxygenase 2 in gastric mucosal lesions and its inhibition by the specific antagonist delays healing in mice. *Gastroenterology*. 1997;112:387–97.

29. Schmassmann A, Peskar BM, Stettler C, Netzer P, Stroff T, Flogerzi B et al. Effects of inhibition of prostaglandin endoperoxide synthase-2 in chronic gastrointestinal ulcer models in rats. *Br J Pharm*. 1998;123:795–804.

30. Hudson N, Balsitis M, Everitt S, Hawkey CJ. Angiogenesis in gastric ulcers: impaired in patients taking non steroidal anti-inflammatory drugs. *Gut*. 1995;37:191–4.

31. Wu KC, Jackson LM, Galvin A, Gray T, Hawkey CJ, Mahida YR. Characterisation of lamina propria lymphocytes, macrophages and myofibroblasts migrating out of human gastric mucosa denuded of epithelial cells. *Gastroenterology*. 1998;114: A1191:G4871.

32. Hull MA, Hewett PW, Brough JL, Hawkey CJ. Isolation and culture of human gastric endothelial cells. *Gastroenterology*. 1996;111:1230–40.

33. Mahida YR, Beltinger J, Makh S, Goke M, Gray T, Podolsky DK et al. Adult human colonic subepithelial myofibroblasts express extracellular matrix proteins and cyclooxygenase-1 and -2. *Am J Physiol*. 1997;273:G1341–G1348.

34. Thun MJ, Namboodiri MM, Calle EE, Flanders WD, Heath CV Jr. Aspirin use and risk of fatal cancer. *Cancer Res*. 1993;53:1322–7.

35. Gridley G, McLaughlin JK, Ekbom A, Klareskog L, Adami HO, Hacker DG et al. Incidence of cancer among patients with rheumatoid arthritis. *J Natl Cancer Inst*. 1993;85:307–11.

36. Logan RFA, Little J, Hawtin PG, Hardcastle JD. Effect of aspirin and non steroidal anti-inflammatory drugs on colorectal adenomas: Case control study of subjects participating in the Nottingham faecal occult blood screening programme. *Br Med J*. 1993;307:285–9.

37. Coffey RJ, Hawkey CJ, Damstrup L, Graves-Deal R, Cunningham GR, Dempsey P et al. Epidermal growth factor receptor-mediated nuclear targeting of COX-2 and basolateral release of prostaglandins linked to cellular proliferation in polarizing colon cancer cells. *Proc Natl Acad Sci USA*. 1997;94:657–62.

38. Serhan CN. Signalling fat controller. *Nature*. 1996;384:23–4.

39. Sano H, Kawahito Y, Wilder RL, Hashiramoto A, Mukai S, Asai K et al. Expression of cyclooxygenase-1 and -2 in human colorectal cancer. *Cancer Res*. 1995;55:3785–9.

9

Management of non-steroidal anti-inflammatory drug-related gastrointestinal mucosal injury

C.-C. TSENG AND M. M. WOLFE

Beginning with the introduction of aspirin, non-steroidal anti-inflammatory drugs (NSAIDs) have become one of the most commonly used medications. It is estimated that more than 1% of the American population uses them on a daily basis[1], and over 35 million NSAID prescriptions and billions of over-the-counter preparations are sold annually in the USA[2]. Although NSAIDs are generally well tolerated, their use is frequently limited by adverse gastrointestinal (GI) effects, ranging from dyspepsia to serious complications, such as bleeding or perforation from gastroduodenal ulcers. In 1984, the Center for Disease Control reported that 100,000 to 200,000 hospitalizations and 10,000 to 20,000 deaths occurred annually in the USA due to the GI side effect of NSAIDs.

PATHOGENESIS OF NSAID-INDUCED GI DAMAGE

Although NSAIDs are commonly known for producing gastroduodenal ulcers, they are capable of inducing widespread injury throughout the entire GI tract and liver. NSAID-induced oesophageal injury has been reported infrequently, and most reports have described pill oesophagitis associated with the ingestion of these acidic compounds[3]. Recently, a protein- and blood-losing enteropathy in individuals receiving chronic NSAID therapy has been reported and was attributed to the development of iron deficiency and hypoalbuminaemia. The cause of this enteropathy is unknown and may include direct vascular injury from NSAIDs, prostaglandin (PG) depletion, and bacterial invasion of the damaged mucosa.

Colonic damage from NSAID use, although less common than small intestinal injury, has been reported. Lanas et al. recently found that approximately 35%

of NSAID-induced GI bleeding actually occurred below the ligament of Treitz[4]. The spectrum of injury ranges from colitis resembling inflammatory bowel disease to colonic perforation and bleeding. Diaphragm-like strictures of the distal small intestine, caecum, and ascending colon have also been associated with the use of NSAIDs. Despite their deleterious effects in the colon, sulindac and other NSAIDs have been reported to induce a partial regression of colorectal adenomas in individuals with familial adenomatous polyposis by virtue of their inhibitory effects on cellular proliferation[5].

Damage to the gastroduodenal mucosa results from both the topical and systemic effects of NSAIDs. The topical effects involve both direct and indirect mechanisms. In the presence of highly acidic gastric contents, non-ionized lipophilic NSAIDs are easily absorbed and migrate through the gastric mucus to the surface epithelium, where they are dissociated into the ionized form, resulting in H^+ ion trapping[6]. In addition, NSAIDs reduce the hydrophobicity of the gastric mucosa and render the surface epithelium susceptible to injury by gastric acid[7]. Indirectly, mucosal erosion may also result from duodenogastric reflux of bile containing active NSAID metabolites[2].

Although topical damage caused by NSAIDs contributes significantly to the development of gastroduodenal mucosal injury, the systemic effects of these agents may play the predominant role. In fact, NSAID-induced gastroduodenal injury occurs with equal frequency using enteric-coated preparations, cutaneous gels, and following either rectal or parenteral administration[8,9]. Furthermore, prodrugs such as sulindac that exhibit their effects only after metabolic transformation into an active compound have been associated with gastroduodenal ulceration. One mechanism that has been shown to contribute to the systemic effect of NSAIDs is a decrease in the mucosal synthesis of PGs[10]. PGs play an important role in stimulating several components of the normal defensive properties of the gastroduodenal mucosa as well as in reducing acid secretion (Table 1).

PGs are derived from arachidonic acid, a phospholipid component present in cell membranes, by the action of phospholipase A_2. Arachidonic acid is converted to PGs or leukotrienes by the cyclooxygenase (COX) and 5-lipoxygenase pathways, respectively[11]. Recently, two related, but distinct, COX isoenzymes, COX-1 and COX-2, have been demonstrated in mammalian cells[12]. Each enzyme is encoded by a separate gene and exhibits a discrete tissue-specific expression[13].

Table 1 Protective properties of the gastroduodenal mucosa

Enhanced mucus secretion
Increased bicarbonate secretion
Increased mucosal blood flow
Enhanced intercellular tight junctions
Decreased transmembrane hydrogen ion permeation
Increased epithelial restitution

Under physiological conditions, COX-1 is expressed constitutively and functions as a 'housekeeping' enzyme in most tissues, including gastric mucosa. The expression of COX-2, especially in macrophages and synovial cells, is induced by inflammation or mitogen stimulation[13]. It has thus been suggested that the anti-inflammatory properties of NSAIDs are mediated through the inhibition of COX-2, whereas untoward effects occur as a result of effects on COX-1[13]. Although ample evidence supports the role of PGs in NSAID-mediated GI injury, recent studies show that COX-1 knockout mice do not develop gastric ulcers spontaneously, suggesting that other mechanisms may also be involved[14]. McCafferty et al.[15] reported that NSAIDs induce vascular endothelial injury by an increase in the number of neutrophils adhering to the vascular endothelium of the gastric microcirculation. These effects occur as a result of an increase in the expression of intercellular adhesion molecule-1 and in the liberation of oxygen-derived free radicals and proteases[15].

RISK FACTORS FOR NSAID GASTRODUODENOPATHY

Although the overall risk of developing a serious GI complication is three times greater in NSAID users than in non-users[16], the presence of upper GI symptoms is an unreliable marker for the presence of gastroduodenal mucosal injury. In the Aspirin Myocardial Infarction Study, only 5% of those with dyspepsia were found to have ulcers[17]. Another study reported that 58% of individuals hospitalized for NSAID-related GI haemorrhage displayed no antecedent symptoms compared with 25% of those who presented with haemorrhage without a prior history of NSAID use[17]. It is thus useful if risk factors can be utilized to identify subgroups of NSAID users who are at particularly high risk for developing complications.

While no subgroup of patients is free from developing NSAID-related ulcers or complications, several factors increase an individual's risk (Table 2). The combined use of a corticosteroid and NSAID has been shown to induce GI

Table 2 Risk factors for development of NSAID-related ulcers

Definite
  Age >60
  Prior history of ulcer
  Concomitant corticosteroid therapy
  Multiple NSAIDs
  Short duration of therapy (<2 weeks)
  Serious systemic illness

Possible
  Concomitant *H. pylori* infection
  Smoking
  Alcohol

complications more than ten times more often than an NSAID alone[18], even though there is no definite association between the use of corticosteroids and the development of ulcers. Advanced age represents another significant risk for NSAID-associated complications, with a 5.6-fold increment in persons over 70 years old[19]. Previous reports on gender-related difference in NSAID-related gastroduodenopathy probably reflect an increase in the use of these medications among women.

Other important risk factors for the development of NSAID-related ulcers and complications include a prior history of gastroduodenal ulcer disease[16]. Whether or not a history of *Helicobacter pylori*-related ulcers increases the risk of NSAID-associated complications is presently unknown. In a group of *H. pylori* infected individuals, Chan et al. recently reported a significant decrease in naproxen-induced ulcers in individuals whose *H. pylori* infection was eradicated[20]. Whether screening for *H. pylori* infection should be recommended prior to the institution of NSAID therapy warrants further investigation.

Although all NSAIDs possess the capacity to induce GI injury, several studies have reported a greater risk of complications with piroxicam and a relatively lower risk with the use of ibuprofen. In addition, the risk of complications is proportional to the dose of NSAID given[21] and decreases inversely with the duration of therapy[16]. Therefore, contrary to popular belief, those at greatest risk would appear to be the elderly who might require high-dose NSAID therapy for a short period of time or who might use them intermittently.

TREATMENT OF NSAID-ASSOCIATED DYSPEPSIA

Dyspeptic symptoms including heartburn, anorexia, abdominal pain or distention have frequently been reported, and in large epidemiological studies approximately 5%–20% of patients taking NSAIDs had these symptoms[22]. In a prospective, double-blind European study to evaluate the effectiveness of H_2 receptor antagonists in treating NSAID-related dyspeptic symptoms, 72% of patients receiving 400 mg twice daily of cimetidine reported resolution of their symptoms, while only 49% of those receiving placebo were symptom free[23]. Van Groenendael et al. also reported improved symptomatic remission with ranitidine 150 mg twice daily compared to placebo (26% vs 6%)[24]. Recently, Taha et al. have shown that famotidine 20 or 40 mg twice daily significantly reduced abdominal pain in arthritis patients receiving NSAIDs by 36.6% and 43.3%, respectively[25]. These studies provide evidence for the beneficial effects of H_2 receptor antagonists in the relief of dyspeptic symptoms associated with NSAIDs, and it would thus be reasonable to recommend their use in those individuals.

TREATMENT OF NSAID-ASSOCIATED ULCERS

Due to the inability of abdominal symptoms to reliably predict the presence of NSAID-related gastroduodenal ulcer, the optimal treatment for patients with ulcers should include the discontinuation of potentially aggravating factors. Non-toxic analgesics such as paracetamol should be substituted for NSAIDs when possible, and in patients with inflammatory arthritides, methotrexate, hydroxychloroquine, azathioprine, sulphasalazine, D-penicillamine, corticosteroids and gold preparations have been advocated as alternative treatments. If NSAID therapy is discontinued, treatment aimed at healing the acute ulcer can be instituted with one of several agents, as discussed below. Lancaster-Smith et al. have reported 95% gastric ulcer healing with ranitidine 150 mg twice daily in patients whose NSAID therapy has been discontinued[26]. Thus, the efficacy of H_2 receptor antagonists in healing ulcers when NSAIDs are discontinued compares favourably to those with 'idiopathic' peptic ulcers. Nevertheless, in a majority of patients, the continuation of NSAIDs is necessary for pain relief.

Sucralphate
Sucralphate, a basic aluminium salt of sucrose octasulphate, is effective in the treatment and prophylaxis of duodenal ulcers and appears to be as effective as H_2 antagonists in the healing of gastric ulcers[27]. Likewise, sucralphate heals duodenal ulcers as effectively as H_2 antagonists whether or not NSAIDs are continued[27]. However, this agent has no proven benefit in the treatment of gastric ulcers.

Prostaglandins
PGs exhibit their therapeutic effects by enhancing mucosal defensive properties and at higher doses by inhibiting gastric acid secretion[28]. Although they are effective in preventing NSAID-induced gastroduodenal mucosal injury, their role in the treatment of NSAID-associated ulcers is unclear. Recently, the efficacy of misoprostol in healing NSAID-associated gastroduodenal ulcers was compared to omeprazole in a double-blind study of 935 individuals who had ulcers or more than 10 erosions in the stomach or duodenum[29]. The rates of successful treatment at eight weeks were similar in patients receiving either 20 or 40 mg of omeprazole or 200 µg four times a day of misoprostol (76%, 75% and 71% improvement, respectively). Omeprazole, as expected, was better tolerated than misoprostol. A detailed analysis of the data indicated that healing rates among patients with gastroduodenal ulcers were higher with omeprazole, whereas misoprostol healed erosions better.

H_2 Receptor Antagonists
The efficacy of H_2 receptor antagonists in the treatment of NSAID-related ulcers has not been extensively assessed. A number of open, uncontrolled, non-randomized studies[30] and prospective, randomized studies[31] suggest that treatment with conventional doses of H_2 receptor antagonists for six to 12 weeks results in healing of approximately 75% (50%–88%) of gastric ulcers and 87% (67%–100%) of duodenal ulcers despite the continued use of NSAIDs. When NSAIDs are continued, healing appears to be delayed and is largely dependent on the initial ulcer size. O'Laughlin et al. reported a 90% healing rate of small

gastric ulcers (less than 5 mm in diameter) after an eight-week course of cimetidine treatment, whereas only 25% of ulcers greater than 5 mm in diameter healed[32]. Extending therapy for an additional 6–26 months healed 86% of large ulcers despite continued NSAID use.

Proton Pump Inhibitors

In addition to the topical effects of NSAIDs, gastric acid appears to play an important role in the pathogenesis of NSAID-associated ulcers. In a multicentre trial, Walan et al.[33] compared the efficacy of omeprazole (20 mg or 40 mg per day) and ranitidine (150 mg twice daily) in the treatment of gastric ulcers in patients who continued taking NSAIDs. Gastric ulcer healing rates at four weeks were 81% in the group receiving 40 mg of omeprazole, 61% in patients treated with 20 mg of omeprazole and 32% in those receiving ranitidine. The corresponding healing rates after eight weeks were 95%, 82% and 53%, respectively. A recent study in a group of 541 patients also demonstrated the superiority of omeprazole over ranitidine in the treatment of NSAID-related gastroduodenal ulcers[34]. In this group of individuals, ulcer healing rates at eight weeks were 79% in those receiving 40 mg of omeprazole, 80% with 20 mg omeprazole, and 63% with ranitidine. Another study by Agrawal et al.[35] compared the efficacy of lansoprazole and ranitidine in the healing of gastric ulcers greater than 0.5 cm in diameter in patients continuing NSAID therapy. After eight weeks, ulcers were healed in 57% of the individuals receiving ranitidine, while healing rates were 73% and 75% in those treated with lansoprazole 15 mg and 30 mg, respectively. These observations suggest that proton pump inhibitors (PPIs) possess the capacity to heal gastroduodenal ulcers at an accelerated rate whether or not NSAIDs are continued.

PROPHYLAXIS OF NSAID-ASSOCIATED GASTRODUODENOPATHY

Due to the significant rate of serious NSAID-related GI complications, recent efforts have been directed at the prevention of mucosal injury induced by NSAIDs. As discussed previously, the best way to eliminate this risk is to avoid the use of NSAIDs and substitute a non-toxic agent. Salsalate, a non-acetylated salicylate, which does not inhibit PG synthesis or induce gastroduodenal injury, can be used as an anti-inflammatory agent. Nevertheless, in a majority of patients, the use of NSAIDs is preferred. Thus, two strategies have been employed to enhance the safety profile of NSAIDs: the use of concomitant medication to protect the gastroduodenal mucosa from NSAID injury and the development of safer anti-inflammatory agents.

Sucralphate

The precise mechanism of mucosal protection by sucralphate has not been elucidated. Sucralphate has been shown by Caldwell et al. to reduce gastroduodenal mucosal injury associated with NSAID use[36]. However, Agrawal et al.[37] reported no significant beneficial effect of sucralphate in the prevention of gastric ulcers in osteoarthritis patients receiving NSAID therapy.

H_2 Receptor Antagonists

Two placebo-controlled, prospective studies investigated the protective effect of ranitidine in arthritis patients receiving concomitant NSAID therapy[38,39]. An eight-week course of treatment with ranitidine 150 mg twice daily proved to be effective in preventing duodenal ulcers, with rates of 0% and 1.5% in the two studies, compared to 8% in placebo-treated patients. In contrast, ranitidine was ineffective in preventing gastric ulcers in both studies. Nevertheless, Taha et al. recently reported a beneficial effect of high-dose famotidine (40 mg twice daily) in preventing both gastric and duodenal ulcers in arthritis patients receiving NSAIDs for 24 weeks[25]. Although H_2 receptor antagonists appear to be effective in reducing NSAID-related ulcers and dyspeptic symptoms, Singh et al. recently found that asymptomatic rheumatoid arthritis patients receiving H_2 receptor antagonists had a significantly higher risk for developing GI complications than those not taking these drugs[40]. Thus, the routine use of H_2 receptor antagonists in the prevention of NSAID-associated ulcers cannot be recommended.

Proton Pump Inhibitors

Although PPIs have been demonstrated to heal gastroduodenal ulcers at an accelerated rate in NSAIDs users, few studies have systematically examined their capacity to protect gastroduodenal mucosa from NSAIDs injury. Oddsson et al. found that omeprazole was effective in reducing naproxen-induced mucosal injury by 40% in the stomach and by 90% in the duodenum in a group of volunteers[41]. In another study, Scheiman et al. reported that omeprazole completely protected the duodenal mucosa from aspirin-induced injury and reduced the severity of aspirin-associated gastric mucosal damage by 45%[42]. More recently, Yeomans et al. compared omeprazole and H_2 receptor antagonists in the prevention of gastroduodenal ulcers in individuals in whom NSAID therapy could not be discontinued. A group of 432 patients were randomly assigned to maintenance treatment with either 20 mg of omeprazole or 150 mg twice daily of ranitidine[34]. At the end of six months, 72% of patients on omeprazole were in remission compared to 59% on ranitidine. Another recent study compared the efficacy of omeprazole and misoprostol in preventing ulcer recurrence in patients continuing NSAID therapy[29]. In this double-blind, placebo-controlled study, 732 patients were randomly administered either placebo, 20 mg of omeprazole, or 200 µg twice daily of misoprostol as maintenance therapy. At six months, duodenal ulcers were detected in 12% and 10% of those treated with placebo and misoprostol, respectively, while only 3% of those treated with omeprazole developed a duodenal ulcer. Gastric ulcer relapse occurred in 32%, 10% and 13% of the individuals receiving placebo, misoprostol, and omeprazole, respectively (Figure 1)[29]. Although the misoprostol dose was lower than that used in other trials, these

Figure 1 Results of the OMNIUM study, a randomized, double-blind, placebo-controlled trial that compared the ability of misoprostol 200 μg twice daily and omeprazole (OMP) 20 mg daily administered for 6 months to prevent the development of NSAID-induced gastric ulcers (GU) and duodenal ulcers (DU). Data adapted from reference 29.

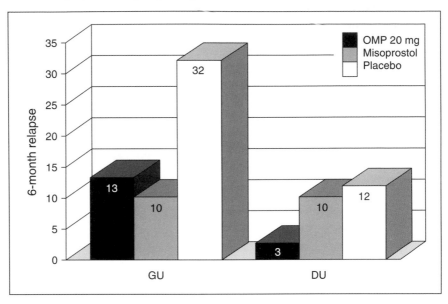

studies suggest that omeprazole is an effective form of therapy for maintaining patients in remission during continued NSAID use.

Misoprostol

As discussed previously, PGs produce their beneficial effects by enhancing mucosal defence mechanisms, while at higher doses they also inhibit acid secretion. In their initial study, Graham et al. showed that the prevalence of gastric ulcers in osteoarthritis patients who had abdominal pain and were receiving NSAIDs was 1.4% in those concomitantly taking 200 μg four times daily of misoprostol, 5.6% in patients receiving 100 μg four times daily of misoprostol and 21.7% in those receiving placebo[43]. The efficacy of misoprostol in duodenal ulcer prophylaxis was confirmed in another study by Graham et al.[44]. In this group of 638 patients with chronic arthritis, misoprostol significantly reduced the incidence of duodenal ulcers from 4.6% in those taking placebo to 0.6% in those taking misoprostol. Despite the effect of misoprostol in preventing gastroduodenal ulcers, a beneficial effect in improving dyspeptic symptoms was not demonstrated in those studies. Furthermore, diarrhoea developed in 39% of those taking 200 μg of misoprostol. Raskin et al.[45] conducted a study to evaluate the prophylactic efficacy of three different doses of misoprostol (200 μg twice daily, three times daily and four times daily) and concluded that, although lower doses of misoprostol are better tolerated, the drug needs to be taken at least three times a day to provide significant prophylaxis for NSAID-induced gastric ulcers. To assess whether misoprostol could affect the incidence of ulcer complications due to NSAID use, Silverstein et al.[46] conducted the MUCOSA (Misoprostol Ulcer Complication Outcomes Safety Assessment) trial. A 40% reduction in overall complications from NSAID-associated ulcers was observed in those taking 200 μg four times daily of misoprostol, although 42% of those receiving misoprostol withdrew from the study due to diarrhoea.

The results of all these trials indicate that although misoprostol is a highly effective form of therapy for preventing NSAID-induced ulcers, and is the only drug approved by the US Food and Drug Administration for prophylaxis against NSAID-related gastroduodenal ulcers, it is associated with a significant number of adverse effects. In addition to diarrhoea and abdominal pain, another significant side effect of misoprostol is increased uterine contractility that can lead to spontaneous abortion, and it is therefore contraindicated in women of childbearing age who are sexually active.

The Use of Safer NSAIDs

Several modifications in the formulation of NSAIDs have been introduced to reduce their toxicity. Recent surveillance and endoscopic studies have confirmed a lower incidence of gastroduodenal mucosal injury associated with the use of nabumetone, etodolac, and meloxicam[47] (Figure 2). Etodolac and meloxicam preferentially inhibit COX-2, with little effect on COX 1, which appears to account for their improved safety profile. These data are consistent with the hypothesis that the preferential inhibition of COX-2 may improve the tolerability and safety of NSAIDs[48].

Figure 2 Postmarketing surveillance of the incidence of ulcer complications (perforations, ulcerations and bleeding – PUBs) in patients taking meloxicam, a preferential COX-2 inhibitor, compared with piroxicam, diclofenac, and naproxen. Data are compared by age (<65 and >65 years) and are adapted from reference 47.

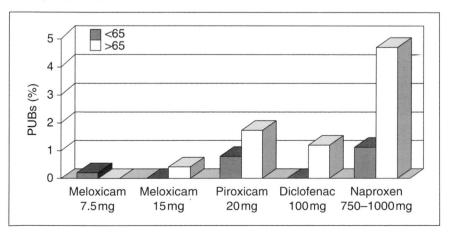

Table 3 Recommendations for management of NSAID-associated gastroduodenal mucosal injury

Clinical presentation	Recommendation
Dyspepsia	Empirical H_2 receptor antagonist (e.g. cimetidine 400 mg bid, ranitidine/nizatidine 150 mg bid, or famotidine 20 mg bid)
Active ulcer	NSAID discontinued: H_2 receptor antagonist or proton pump inhibitor
	NSAID continued: proton pump inhibitor
Maintenance therapy	Co-administration of proton pump inhibitor
	Co-administration of misoprostol (at least 200 μg tid), or NSAIDs with improved safety profile (e.g. nabumetone, etodolac or meloxicam)

bid=twice daily; tid=three times a day

FUTURE DEVELOPMENT OF SAFER NSAIDS

Several compounds have been developed to produce safer NSAIDs. These include highly selective COX-2 inhibitors, nitric oxide releasing NSAIDs, and NSAIDs pre-associated with zwitterionic phospholipids. Although initial studies indicate that these compounds offer significant promise in reducing NSAID toxicities, their potential use awaits further clinical investigation. Furthermore, trefoil peptides and basic fibroblast growth factor may eventually prove clinically useful in protecting the mucosa against NSAID-induced injury.

SUMMARY

The current approach to patients taking NSAIDs is summarized in Table 3. NSAID-associated dyspeptic symptoms are common and can be managed empirically with an H_2 receptor antagonist. Treatment of established gastroduodenal ulcers is best accomplished by withholding the offending drugs. PPIs appear to heal ulcers at the same rate whether or not NSAID therapy is continued. After the ulcer is healed and if NSAID therapy must be continued, prophylaxis is best accomplished by the concomitant use of PPIs or misoprostol (at least 200 μg three times a day), together with the use of a classical NSAID or one that preferentially inhibits COX-2. Whether preferential COX-2 inhibitors also exhibit improved GI tolerability (for example, for dyspepsia) remains to be seen.

REFERENCES

1. McCarthy DM. Nonsteroidal antiinflammatory drug-induced ulcers: management by traditional therapies. *Gastroenterology*. 1989;96:662–74.
2. Lichtenstein DR, Syngal S, Wolfe MM. Nonsteroidal antiinflammatory drugs and the gastrointestinal tract. *Arthritis Rheum*. 1995;38:5–18.
3. Minoch A, Greenbaum DS. Pill-esophagitis caused by nonsteroidal antiinflammatory drugs. *Am J Gastroenterol*. 1991;86:1086–9.

4. Lanas A, Sekar MC, Hirshowitz BI. Objective evidence of aspirin use in both ulcer and nonulcer upper and lower gastrointestinal bleeding. *Gastroenterology.* 1992;103:862–9.

5. Logan RF, Little J, Hawtin PG, Hardcastle JD. Effect of aspirin and non-steroidal antiinflammatory drugs on colorectal adenomas: case-control study of subjects participating in the Nottingham faecal occult blood screening programme. *Br Med J.* 1993;307:285–9.

6. Somasundaram S, Hayllar H, Rafi S, Wrigglesworth JM, Macpherson AJ, Bjarnason I. The biochemical basis of non-steroidal anti-inflammatory drug-induced damage to the gastrointestinal tract: a review and a hypothesis. *Scand J Gastroenterol.* 1995;30:289–99.

7. Lichtenberger LM. The hydrophobic barrier properties of gastrointestinal mucus. *Annu Rev Physiol.* 1995;57:565–83.

8. Henry D, Dobson A, Turner C. Variability in the risk of major gastrointestinal complications from nonaspirin nonsteroidal anti-inflammatory drugs. *Gastroenterology.* 1993;10:1078–88.

9. Zimmerman J, Siguencia J, Tsvang E. Upper gastrointestinal hemorrhage associated with cutaneous application of diclofenac gel. *Am J Gastroenterol.* 1995;90:2032–4.

10. Soll AH, Weinstein WM, Kurata J, McCarthy D. Nonsteroidal antiinflammatory drugs and peptic ulcer disease. *Ann Intern Med.* 1991;114:307–19.

11. Schoen RT, Vender RJ. Mechanisms of nonsteroidal antiinflammatory drug-induced gastric damage. *Am J Med.* 1989;86:449–59.

12. Masferrer JL, Seibert K, Zweifel B, Needleman P. Endogenous glucocorticoids regulate an inducible cyclooxygenase enzyme. *Proc Natl Acad Sci USA.* 1992;89:3917–21.

13. Crofford LJ. COX-1 and COX-2 tissue expression: implications and predictions. *J Rheumatol.* 1997;24(suppl 49):15 9.

14. Langenbach R, Morham SG, Tiano HF, Loftin CD, Ghanayem BI, Chulada PC et al. Prostaglandin synthase 1 gene disruption in mice reduces arachidonic acid-induced inflammation and indomethacin-induced gastric ulceration. *Cell.* 1995;83:483–92.

15. McCafferty DM, Granger DN, Wallace JL. Indomethacin-induced gastric injury and leukocyte adherence in arthritic versus healthy rats. *Gastroenterology.* 1995;109:1173 80.

16. Gabriel SE, Jaakkimainen L, Bombardier C. Risk for serious gastrointestinal complications related to use of nonsteroidal anti-inflammatory dugs: a meta-analysis. *Ann Intern Med.* 1991;115:787–96.

17. Aspirin Myocardial Infarction Study Research Group. A randomized, controlled trial of aspirin in persons recovered from myocardial infarction. *J Am Med Assoc.* 1980;243:661–9.

18. Piper JM, Ray WA, Daugherty JR, Griffin MR. Corticosteroid use and peptic ulcer disease: role of nonsteroidal antiinflammatory drugs. *Ann Intern Med.* 1991;114:735–40.

19. Griffin MR, Ray WA, Schaffner W. Nonsteroidal antiinflammatory drug use and death from peptic ulcer in elderly persons. *Ann Intern Med.* 1988;109:359–63.

20. Chan FKL, Sung JJY, Chung SCS, To KF, Yung MY, Leung VK. Randomized trial of eradication of Helicobacter pylori before non-steroidal antiinflammatory drug therapy to prevent peptic ulcers. *Lancet.* 1997;350:975–9.

21. Griffin MR, Ray WA, Schaffner W. Nonsteroidal antiinflammatory drug use and increased risk for peptic ulcer disease in elderly persons. *Ann Intern Med.* 1991;114:257–63.

22. Langman MJS. Epidemiologic evidence of the association between peptic ulceration and antiinflammatory drug use. *Gastroenterology.* 1989;96:640–6.

23. Bijlsma JW. Treatment of NSAID-induced gastrointestinal lesions with cimetidine: An international multicenter collaborative study. *Aliment Pharmacol Ther.* 1988;2S:85–95.

24. Van Groenendael JHLM, Markusse HM, Dijkmans BAC, Breedveld FC. The effect of ranitidine on NSAID related dyspeptic symptoms with and without peptic ulcer disease of patients with rheumatoid arthritis and osteoarthritis. *Clin Rheumatol.* 1996;15:450–6.

25. Taha AS, Hudson N, Hawkey CJ, Swannell AJ, Trye PN, Cottrell J et al. Famotidine for the prevention of gastric and duodenal ulcers caused by nonsteroidal antiinflammatory drugs. *N Engl J Med.* 1996;334:1435–9.
26. Lancaster-Smith MJ, Jaderberg ME, Jackson DA. Ranitidine in the treatment of non-steroidal antiinflammatory drug associated gastric and duodenal ulcers. *Gut.* 1990;32:252–5.
27. McCarthy DM. Sucralfate. *N Engl J Med.* 1991;325:1017–25.
28. Wolfe MM, Soll AH. The physiology of gastric acid secretion. *N Engl J Med.* 1988;319:1707–15.
29. Hawkey CJ, Karrasch JA, Szczepanski L, Walker DG, Barkun A, Swannell AJ et al. Omeprazole compared with misoprostol for ulcers associated with nonsteroidal anti-inflammatory drugs. *N Engl J Med.* 1998;338:727–34.
30. Croker JR, Cotten PB, Boyle AC, Kinsella P. Cimetidine for peptic ulcer in patients with arthritis. *Ann Rheum Dis.* 1980;39:275–8.
31. Davies J, Collins AJ, Dixon ASJ. The influence of cimetidine on peptic ulcer in patients with arthritis taking antiinflammatory drugs. *Br J Rheumatol.* 1986;25:54–8.
32. O'Laughlin JC, Silvoso GK, Ivey KJ. Resistance to medical therapy of gastric ulcers in rheumatic disease patients taking aspirin. *Dig Dis Sci.* 1982;27:976–80.
33. Walan A, Bader JP, Classen M, Lamers CB, Piper DW, Rutgersson K et al. Effect of omepra-zole and ranitidine on ulcer healing and relapse rates in patients with benign gastric ulcer. *N Engl J Med.* 1989;320:69–75.
34. Yeomans ND, Tulassay Z, Juhász L, Rácz I, Howard JM, van Rensburg CJ et al. A comparison of omeprazole with ranitidine for ulcers associated with nonsteroidal anti-inflammatory drugs. *N Engl J Med.* 1998;338:719–26.
35. Agrawal N, Safadi M, Wruble L, Karvois D, Greski-Rose P, Huang B. Effectiveness of lansoprazole in the healing of NSAID-induced gastric ulcers in patients continuing to take NSAIDs. *Gastroenterology.* 1998;114:A52.
36. Caldwell JR, Roth SH, Wu WC, Semble EL, Castell DO, Heller MD et al. Sucralfate treat-ment of nonsteroidal antiinflammatory drug-induced gastrointestinal symptoms and mucosal damage. *Am J Med.* 1987;83(suppl 3B):74–82.
37. Agrawal NM, Roth S, Graham DY, White RH, Germain B, Brown JA et al. Misoprostol compared with sucralfate in the prevention of nonsteroidal antiinflammatory drug-induced gastric ulcer: a randomized, controlled trial. *Ann Intern Med.* 1991;115:911–3.
38. Robinson MG, Griffin JW, Bowers J, Kogan FJ, Kogut DG, Lauza FL et al. Effect of ranitidine on gastroduodenal mucosal damage induced by nonsteroidal antiinflammatory drugs. *Dig Dis Sci.* 1989;34:424–8.
39. Ehsanullah RSB, Page MC, Tildesly G, Wood JR. Prevention of gastrointestinal damage induced by nonsteroidal antiinflammatory drugs: controlled trial of ranitidine. *Br Med J.* 1988;297:1017–21.
40. Singh G, Ramey DR, Morfeld D, Shi H, Hatoum HT, Fries JF. Gastrointestinal tract com-plications of nonsteroidal antiinflammatory drug treatment in rheumatoid arthritis: A prospective observational cohort study. *Arch Intern Med.* 1996;156:1530–6.
41. Oddsson E, Gudjonsson H, Thjodleifsson B. Comparison between ranitidine and omepra-zole for protection against gastroduodenal damage caused by naproxen. *Scand J Gastroenterol.* 1992;27:1045–8.
42. Scheiman JM, Behler EM, Loeffler KM, Elta GH. Omeprazole ameliorates aspirin-induced gastroduodenal injury. *Dig Dis Sci.* 1994;39:97–103.
43. Graham DY, Agrawal NM, Roth SH. Prevention of NSAID-induced gastric ulcer with misoprostol: multicenter, double-blind, placebo-controlled trial. *Lancet.* 1988;2:1277–80.

44. Graham DY, White RH, Moreland LW, Schubert TT, Katz R, Jaszewski R et al. Duodenal and gastric ulcer prevention with misoprostol in arthritis patients taking NSAIDs. *Ann Intern Med*. 1993;119:257–62.

45. Raskin JB, White RH, Jackson JE, Weaver AL, Tindall EA, Lies RB et al. Misoprostol dosage for the prevention of nonsteroidal antiinflammatory drug-induced gastric and duodenal ulcers: a comparison of three regimens. *Ann Intern Med*. 1995;123:344–50.

46. Silverstein FE, Graham DY, Senior JR, Davies HW, Struthers BJ, Bittman RM et al. Misoprostol reduces serious gastrointestinal complications in patient with rheumatoid arthritis receiving nonsteroidal antiinflammatory drugs: a randomized, double-blind, placebo-controlled trial. *Ann Intern Med*. 1995;123:241–9.

47. Distel M, Mueller C, Bluhmki E, Fries J. Safety of meloxicam: a global analysis of clinical trials. *Br J Rheumatol*. 1996;35(suppl 1):68–77.

48. Vane JR, Botting RM. Mechanism of action of antiinflammatory drugs. *Scand J Rheumatol*. 1996;25(suppl 102):9–21.

10

Avoidance of renal side effects of non-steroidal anti-inflammatory drugs: value of selective cyclooxygenase-2 inhibition

D. O. STICHTENOTH AND J. C. FRÖLICH

After the gastrointestinal tract, the kidney is the most frequent target of adverse effects of non-steroidal anti-inflammatory drugs (NSAIDs). The unwanted renal effects of NSAIDs can be divided into three categories: (1) Renal side effects of NSAIDs due to inhibition of prostanoid synthesis. Most of the unwanted renal effects of NSAIDs are related to this mechanism, including reduction in renal blood flow (RBF), glomerular filtration rate (GFR), sodium retention and hyperkalacmia[1]. (2) Analgesic nephropathy. Habitual use of NSAIDs and non-NSAID analgesics can cause analgesic nephropathy, which is characterized by a slowly developing process leading to the characteristic papillary necrosis. For NSAIDs, the chronic reduction in perfusion of the renal medulla is the most likely to lead to ischaemic damage[1]. For the non-NSAID analgesics, the mechanism of damage is unknown[2]. (3) Interstitial nephritis. Besides the NSAIDs, many drugs can cause interstitial nephritis, which has been postulated to be a cell-mediated immune response[3].

The incidence of all renal side effects occurs in up to 18% of NSAID-treated patients; severe renal side effects with clinically apparent symptoms occur in 1% of individuals taking NSAIDs[4]. The absolute values are high, due to the large exposure to NSAIDs. It is estimated that more than 10% of the population in developed countries are taking NSAIDs intermittently or routinely per year. Moreover, 10% of these patients combine two or more NSAIDs. As a result, 3% of all cases of acute renal failure are caused by NSAIDs and in patients with endstage renal failure NSAIDs are implicated as causal agents in up to 30% of individuals[3,5]. Thus, any effort to avoid the renal side effects of NSAIDs is of great therapeutic importance.

PHYSIOLOGY OF PROSTANOIDS IN THE KIDNEY AND EFFECTS OF NSAIDS

The predominant prostanoids produced in the kidney are prostaglandin (PG) E_2, prostacyclin (PGI_2) and, to a lesser degree, $PGF_{2\alpha}$[6]. PGI_2 is primarily synthesized in the kidney cortex and PGE_2 in the medulla[7]. More detailed analyses of the isolated structures of the kidney have shown that the renal vasculature and glomeruli produce mainly PGI_2, while renomedullary interstitial cells synthesize predominantly PGE_2[8]. Also there is some thromboxane A_2 synthesis, although its function is uncertain[7].

The intrarenal effects of these prostanoids are mediated by G-protein-coupled receptors. It must be emphasized that the occurrence of multiple receptor subtypes and their specific pattern of distribution are responsible for the multiple, and at times apparently opposing, effects of a single prostaglandin[9].

One of the most substantial challenges has been to analyse renal prostanoid production in vivo. Blood levels of prostanoids are unreliable parameters, due to the possibility of platelet activation and irritation of the vascular wall. Thus, urinary PGE_2 excretion reflects renal prostaglandin production. However, in males, seminal fluid may interfere with PGE_2 measurements as it contains high amounts of PGE_2. Furthermore, prostaglandin excretion may depend on the rate of urine flow and its pH, as prostaglandins are weak acids. When these parameters are controlled, measurement of urinary PGE_2 in females is a valid index of renal prostaglandin production in humans[10].

Regulation of Renal Haemodynamics

The first evidence for an effect of prostanoids on RBF stems from the infusion of PGE_1 into the renal artery of dogs, which produced an increase in RBF[11]. Other prostanoids including PGE_2, PGD_2 and PGI_2 were also shown to cause an increase in RBF[12]. Inhibition of cyclooxygenase (COX) by indomethacin in anaesthetized, laparatomized dogs showed a striking reduction of RBF and led to the proposal that prostanoids are responsible for regulation of basal RBF[13]. However, in conscious dogs indomethacin had no effect on RBF[14]. This difference points to the important role of other mediators which, when unopposed by renal prostanoids, cause pronounced vasoconstriction. A wealth of information has now accumulated to suggest that in pathophysiological states prostanoids help to maintain RBF and GFR. This is particularly true for those disorders characterized by a low effective plasma volume: cirrhosis with ascites, heart failure and the nephrotic syndrome, where vasoconstrictor effects of renal nerve activity, catecholamines, angiotensin II and vasopressin play an important role. Accordingly, indomethacin causes a striking decrease in GFR in patients with these diseases[15-17]. Other conditions in which inhibition of prostanoid synthesis reduces GFR and can induce acute renal failure include Bartter's syndrome, chronic renal insufficiency, systemic lupus erythematosus with renal involvement and diuretics or dietary sodium depletion[18].

A further effect of renal prostanoid inhibition with far-reaching consequences is due to medullary blood flow being provided exclusively by the juxtamedullary nephrons. Inhibition of prostanoid synthesis will cause a redistribution of blood flow within the kidney away from the medulla. Thus, prostanoids play a critical role in protecting the renal medulla from ischaemic damage[19]. This may be an important contributing factor to papillary necrosis caused by currently used NSAIDs.

Electrolyte Excretion
Sodium
Infusion of arachidonic acid or PGE_2 causes natriuresis[11]. This effect is coupled with vasodilatation and may be the cause of the natriuresis, presumably by an effect on proximal tubular salt and water reabsorption. Furthermore, the role of antidiuretic hormone (ADH) on sodium transport must be considered. Prostanoids antagonize ADH actions (see below), thus contributing to sodium excretion. However, there is evidence that tubular transport is influenced by prostanoids directly. Microinfusions of ^{22}Na into the distal end of the proximal tubule show that co-infusion of PGE_2 reduces sodium reabsorption[20]. Studies in isolated renal tubule segments demonstrated that PGE_2 inhibits sodium transport out of the cortical collecting tubule[21]. From these studies it can be deduced that prostanoids, most likely PGE_2, reduce sodium reabsorption in a segment beyond the proximal tubule. This prostanoid-dependent inhibition of sodium reabsorption occurs primarily in the juxtamedullary nephrons.

In humans, the evidence of sodium retention following prostanoid suppression is quite convincing. We were able to show that, in patients with postmalignant hypertension on a 100 mEq Na^+-diet, indomethacin 25 mg three times a day readily caused inhibition of renal prostanoid production, sodium retention and weight gain[22]. In normal volunteers sodium retention and weight gain are more difficult to demonstrate[22]. In contrast, in patients with nephrotic syndrome, congestive heart failure or liver cirrhosis, sodium retention is easily observed after prostanoid inhibition and may lead to significant clinical deterioration[15-17].

The simultaneous decrease of RBF, GFR and sodium excretion makes it difficult to localize the site of action of the drugs. However, in most studies sodium retention is more severe than can be explained solely by a reduction in the filtered load, and an increased tubular reabsorption is the only explanation.

Potassium
In the macula densa, PGI_2 and PGE_2 mediate renin release[23,24]. Thus, potassium excretion can be reduced by NSAIDs. Convincingly, we showed that indomethacin completely abrogates the increase in plasma renin activity (PRA) seen within minutes after giving furosemide intravenously to healthy volunteers[22]. In sodium-depleted normal volunteers suppression of PRA by NSAIDs can be observed only

under conditions of inhibited sympathetic drive of renin release by non-selective beta-receptor blockade. Under these conditions, when sodium retention was eliminated by a low sodium diet, renin release could be blocked by indomethacin[25]. Hyperkalaemia is not a common problem in patients with normal renal function, but may become a severe threat to the patient with renal disease, which may by itself cause potassium retention, or when drugs which cause potassium retention, such as potassium-sparing diuretics, are taken simultaneously.

Lithium

Effects of NSAIDs on lithium plasma levels are described in several case reports. We studied this drug interaction in a controlled fashion and showed that plasma lithium concentration increased with indomethacin and diclofenac[18]. This effect is due to a decrease in renal lithium clearance and has been observed with other NSAIDs including oxyphenbutazone and ketoprofen.

Antidiuretic Hormone

PGE_2 and $PGF_{2\alpha}$ attenuate the hydro-osmotic effect of ADH as part of a negative feedback loop, where ADH stimulates renal prostaglandin synthesis[26]. This interaction takes place in the renal medulla and is related to the antidiuretic and not the pressor activity of ADH, because its non-pressor analogue, deamino-8-D-arginine vasopressin, also shows a dose-dependent stimulation of renal prostaglandin synthesis[27]. NSAIDs interrupt this negative feedback mechanism. In hypophysectomized dogs indomethacin or meclofenamate administration produced a powerful increase of urine osmolality in response to ADH[28]. Also, in humans, infusion of hypertonic saline increases urine osmolality and free water reabsorption, and both effects are enhanced by indomethacin[29], showing that endogenous ADH, released in large amounts by hypertonic saline, will become more effective when renal prostanoid production is suppressed.

The mechanism of the interaction between ADH and prostanoids has been studied repeatedly, but no convincing evidence has been forthcoming. Mechanisms which have been discussed include an interaction at the level of cAMP, prostanoid effects on solute concentration in the renal papilla and changes in the intracellular calcium pool, which is required for the action of ADH[18]. From a functional point of view, it is important to recognize that under the maximum influence of ADH virtually no barrier to water reabsorption exists and there is complete equilibrium with the medullary interstitium. Under these conditions inhibition of prostanoid synthesis is still effective and enhances antidiuresis. Thus, an influence on water permeability alone cannot explain the findings.

AVOIDANCE OF NSAID SIDE EFFECTS – SELECTIVE INHIBITION OF COX-2

So far, the efforts which have been made to avoid the side effects of NSAIDs have been unsuccessful or only partially successful. The discovery of two different forms of COX, COX-1 and COX-2, ushered in a new generation of NSAIDs with the promise of fewer side effects. COX-1 is the constitutive enzyme, mediating gastric mucosal protection, platelet aggregation, maintenance of renal function and regulation of blood flow[30]. In contrast, COX-2 is induced in many cells by cytokines, mitogens or bacterial endotoxin, suggesting that in inflammatory reactions enhanced prostanoid production is due to induction of COX-2[30]. This makes COX-2 an outstanding target for therapeutic intervention. It is suggested that a drug with selectivity for COX-2 would inhibit pro-inflammatory prostanoid synthesis while sparing physiological prostanoid synthesis. Thus, this drug should be anti-inflammatory with less or none of the typical NSAID-induced adverse effects[31]. As far as the gastrointestinal tract and platelets are concerned, there is a large body of evidence that selective COX-2 inhibition holds this promise. Knowledge of COX isoenzyme selectivity allows prediction of major therapeutic and side effects of NSAIDs. Thus, a classification of NSAIDs on the basis of their inhibitory activity on COX-1 and COX-2 is suggested[32]:

1. *Selective COX-1 inhibitors*. This category comprises only low-dose acetylsalicylic acid, which selectively inhibits COX-1 in platelets.
2. *Non-selective COX inhibitors*. Most of the current NSAIDs inhibit both COX isoenzymes. They reduce platelet aggregation, resulting in prolonged bleeding time, and cause significant gastrointestinal and renal side effects[32]. They will also interact with antihypertonic drugs and lithium[18]. A subclass of drugs with preference for COX-1, which cause a higher risk of these adverse effects[32], can be identified, e.g. indomethacin.
3. *Selective COX-2 inhibitors*, including non-acetylated salicylates and meloxicam. These drugs have no effect on platelet aggregation[33,34] and fewer adverse effects than non-selective COX inhibitors in equivalent therapeutic doses[32].
4. *Highly selective COX-2 inhibitors* in clinical development, which are expected to have no or minimal typical NSAID-induced side effects.

COX ISOENZYMES IN THE KIDNEY

COX-1 has been found in arteries and arterioles, glomeruli and collecting ducts. Remarkably, no COX-1 has been found in the proximal or distal convoluted tubule, the loop of Henle or macula densa[35]. COX-2 has been detected in low concentrations in the kidneys of accident victims, but no localization has been given[36]. In a recent immunohistochemical study, COX-1 immunoreactive protein was localized in the collecting duct and in interstitial, endothelial and smooth muscle cells[37]. COX-2 was found in endothelial and smooth muscle cells of blood vessels and intraglomerularly in podocytes. No COX isoforms were detected in the macula densa[37]. Thus, prostanoids mediating renin release probably stem from the afferent arterioles and tubular cells.

These findings suggest that COX-2 may be involved to some degree in the regulation of renal perfusion and glomerular haemodynamics. However, human in vivo studies and clinical data suggest that under normal basal conditions COX-2 plays a minor role in the kidney. For example, glucocorticoids inhibit the induction of COX-2. Thus, if COX-2-derived prostanoids were important in the kidney[18], glucocorticoids should have detrimental effects on renal function. However, this has never been shown. Also the quantity of PGE_2 produced by the normal kidney, in man, is not reduced by high doses of glucocorticoids, showing that this is a minor pathway for renal PGE_2 production[38]. The sodium retention seen after glucocorticoid administration is due to their mineralocorticoid effect. Non-acetylated salicylates are selective inhibitors of COX-2[39]. They do not inhibit renal PGE_2 synthesis and do not cause reduction in renal blood flow and GFR, sodium retention, water intoxication or a decrease in renal lithium clearance[18,33].

Animal experimental data supplement these human findings. In a detailed analysis of the distribution of COX enzymes in the rat kidney, Harris et al.[40] reported that under control conditions some COX-2 was present in the cortex, papilla and in medullary interstitial cells, which increased strikingly in the cortex during long-term sodium depletion. The major location of COX-2 was in the macula densa, which is important for the control of renin release. These findings were confirmed in vivo[41]. Indomethacin as well as the highly selective COX-2 inhibitor SC-58125 blocked the furosemide-stimulated PRA in rats on a low sodium diet. Thus, COX-2 may play a dominant role in the control of renin release in the rat kidney. Interestingly, urinary PGE_2 excretion was markedly reduced by indomethacin but unaffected by SC-58125, suggesting that, apart from the macula densa, renal prostanoid production in rats is COX-1-dependent.

EXPERIENCE WITH NEW SELECTIVE COX-2 INHIBITORS

Meloxicam is the best documented new NSAID with up to 75-fold selectivity for COX-2 in vitro[42]. We have demonstrated that in healthy volunteers meloxicam 7.5 mg/day, in contrast to indomethacin in the equivalent anti-inflammatory dosage of 25 mg three times a day, had no effect on platelet aggregation and thromboxane formation, indicating that meloxicam at this dose level is COX-1-sparing in humans in vivo[34]. Interestingly, renal PGE_2 synthesis remained un-affected by meloxicam but was markedly inhibited by indomethacin[34]. Thus it can be concluded that the vast majority of renal PGE_2 is synthesized by COX-1. This is in agreement with the effects of glucocorticoids (see above)[38].

Clinical studies suggest that this selectivity, seen in normal volunteers, trans-lates into a renal-sparing effect. A study in 25 patients with mild renal impair-ment, who were at high risk of renal failure, reported that meloxicam in the maximum recommended dose of 15 mg/day for 28 days did not cause further deterioration of renal function[43]. Also, in patients with chronic cardiac failure, another risk factor for impairment of renal function by NSAIDs, meloxicam 15 mg/day for seven days did not cause any renal side effects or attenuate the diuretic effect of furosemide[44]. Recently, the results of two large-scale, double-blind trials comparing meloxicam 7.5 mg to diclofenac 100 mg slow release and piroxicam 20 mg in patients with osteoarthritis were presented. While meloxicam was equivalent with respect to clinical efficacy, the rate of renal toxicity of meloxicam, measured as an increase of creatinine and urea in serum, was significantly less compared with the non-selective COX-inhibitors[45]. While this shows a much reduced risk of renal problems with meloxicam, it also shows that the drug will not be completely free of renal side effects.

What are the effects of a selective COX-2 inhibitor on renin release in the macula densa? In contrast to the rat, where COX-2 mediates renin release, the human in vitro data did not show which COX isoenzyme was involved. Our previous observation suggested a preformed enzyme[22]. To address this issue, we compared in a randomized cross-over study in healthy volunteers the effects of meloxicam in the COX-1-sparing dosage of 7.5 mg/day in comparison with indomethacin 25 mg three times a day on PRA. We found that meloxicam inhibited the furosemide-stimulated PRA as effectively as indomethacin, suggesting that the COX isoenzyme responsible for renin release in man is COX-2[46]. Thus, hyperkalaemia must be considered as a side effect of COX-2 inhibition.

The selective COX-2 inhibitors approved so far by drug-regulatory authorities show at best a 100-fold selectivity for COX-2. Thus they can exert, in upper therapeutic doses, clinically relevant COX-1 inhibition. The prospect of finding new NSAIDs with a higher selectivity for COX-2 has led to the development of numerous new candidate drugs. The leading drugs of this class are currently celecoxib (SC-58635, Monsanto/Searle) and MK-966 (Merck-Frosst). They possess up to 1000-fold selectivity for COX-2 and are now being tested in phase III trials. While sparing of the gastrointestinal tract and platelets by highly selective COX-2 inhibitors is well documented, the renal safety of these drugs needs to be investigated. Remarkably, there are unpublished reports that even the highly selective COX-2 inhibitors can cause oedema and weight gain. However, the relationship to COX inhibition is unknown. A study on flosulide (CGP28238, formerly Ciba-Geigy, development stopped) showed suppression of PRA in man[47], supporting our findings of COX-2 as the isoenzyme responsible for renin release.

In summary, selective COX-2 inhibition holds the promise of providing drugs which have significantly less renal side effects than existing therapy. This is particularly true for the avoidance of a reduction in GFR/RBF, medullary damage, sodium retention and interactions with antihypertensive drugs and lithium. However, hyperkalaemia has to be considered as a possible remaining typical NSAID side effect.

REFERENCES

1. Schlondorff D. Renal complications of nonsteroidal anti-inflammatory drugs. *Kidney Int.* 1993;44:643–53.

2. De Broe ME, Elseviers MM. Analgesic nephropathy. *N Engl J Med.* 1998;338:446–52.

3. Kleinknecht D. Diseases of the kidney caused by non-steroidal antiinflammatory drugs. In: Stewart JH, editor. *Analgesic and NSAID-Induced Kidney Disease.* Oxford: Oxford University Press; 1993:160–79.

4. Murray MD, Brater DC, Tierney WM, Jui SL, McDonald CJ. Ibuprofen-associated renal impairment in a large general internal medicine practice. *Am J Med Sci.* 1990;299:222–9.

5. Schwarz A, Offermann G, Keller F. Analgesic nephropathy and renal transplantation. *Nephrol Dial Transplant.* 1992;7:427–32.

6. Larsson C, Ämggård E. Regional differences in the formation and metabolism of prostaglandins in the rabbit kidney. *Eur J Pharmacol.* 1973;21:30–6.

7. Whorton AR, Smigel M, Oates JA, Frölich JC. Regional differences in prostaglandin formation by the kidney: Prostacyclin is a major prostaglandin of renal cortex. *Biochim Biophys Acta.* 1978;529:176–80.

8. Garcia-Perez A, Smith WL. Apical-basolateral membrane asymmetry in canine cortical collecting tubule cells: bradykinin, arginine vasopressin, prostaglandin E_2 interrelationships. *J Clin Invest.* 1984;74:63–74.

9. Breyer MD, Jacobson HR, Breyer RM. Functional and molecular aspects of renal prostaglandin receptors. *J Am Soc Nephrol.* 1996;7:8–17.

10. Frölich JC, Wilson TW, Sweetman BJ, Smigel M, Nies AS, Carr K et al. Urinary prostaglandins. Identification and origin. *J Clin Invest.* 1975;55:763–70.

11. Johnston HH, Herzog JP, Lauler DP. Effect of prostaglandin E_1 on renal hemodynamics, sodium and water excretion. *Am J Physiol.* 1967;213:939–46.

12. Lifschitz MD. Prostaglandins and renal blood flow. *Kidney Int.* 1981;19:781–5.

13. Aiken JW, Vane JR. Intrarenal prostaglandin release attenuates the renal vasoconstrictor activity of angiotensin. *J Pharmacol Ther.* 1973;184:678–87.

14. Kirschenbaum MA, Stein JH. Effect of inhibition of prostaglandin synthesis on urinary sodium excretion in conscious dogs. *J Clin Invest.* 1976;57:517–21.

15. Arisz L, Donker AJM, Brentjens JRH, van der Hem GK. The effect of indomethacin on proteinuria and kidney function in the nephrotic syndrome. *Acta Med Scand.* 1976;199:121–5.

16. Walshe JJ, Venuto RC. Acute oliguric renal failure induced by indomethacin: possible mechanism. *Ann Intern Med.* 1979;91:47–9.

17. Antillon M, Cominelli F, Lo S, Maran M, Somberg K, Reynolds T et al. Effects of oral prostaglandins on indomethacin induced renal failure in patients with cirrhosis and ascites. *J Rheumatol.* 1990;17:46–9.

18. Frölich JC, Stichtenoth DO. NSAID: can renal side effects be avoided? In: Vane JR, Botting JH, Botting RM, editors. *Improved Non-Steroid Anti-Inflammatory Drugs: COX-2 Enzyme Inhibitors.* London: Kluwer Academic Publishers, and William Harvey Press; 1996:203–28.

19. Brezis M, Rosen S. Hypoxia of the renal medulla – its implications for disease. *N Engl J Med.* 1995;332:647–55.

20. Kauker ML. Prostaglandin E_2 effect from the luminal side on renal tubular ^{22}Na efflux: tracer microinjection studies. *Proc Soc Exp Biol Med.* 1977;154:274–7.

21. Stokes JB, Kokko JP. Inhibition of sodium transport by prostaglandin E_2 across the isolated, perfused rabbit collecting tubule. *J Clin Invest.* 1977;59:1099–104.

22. Frölich JC, Hollifield JW, Dormois BL, Frölich BL, Seyberth H, Michelakis AM et al. Suppression of plasma renin activity by indomethacin in man. *Circ Res.* 1976;39:447–52.

23. Whorton AR, Misono K, Hollifield J, Frölich JC, Inagami T, Oates JA. Prostaglandins and renin release: I. Stimulation of renin release from rabbit renal cortical slices by PGI_2. *Prostaglandins.* 1977;14:1095–104.

24. Ito S, Carretero OA, Abe K, Beierwaltes WH, Yoshinaga K. Effect of prostanoids on renin release from rabbit isolated afferent arterioles with and without attached macula densa. *Kidney Int*. 1989;35:1138–44.

25. Frölich JC, Hollifield JW, Michelakis AM, Vesper BS, Wilson JP, Shand DG et al. Reduction of plasma renin activity by inhibition of the fatty acid cyclooxygenase in human subjects: independence of sodium retention. *Circ Res*. 1979;44:781–7.

26. Walker LA, Whorton AR, Smigel M, France R, Frölich JC. Antidiuretic hormone increases renal prostaglandin synthesis in vivo. *Am J Physiol*. 1978; 235:F180–F185.

27. Walker LA, Frölich JC. Dose-dependent stimulation of renal prostaglandin synthesis by deamino-8-D-arginine vasopressin in rats with hereditary diabetes insipidus. *J Pharmacol Exp Ther*. 1981;271:87–91.

28. Anderson RJ, Berl T, McDonald KM, Schrier RW. Evidence for an in vivo antagonism between vasopressin and prostaglandin in the mammalian kidney. *J Clin Invest*. 1975;56:420–6.

29. Kramer HJ, Backer A, Hinzen S, Dusing R. Effects of inhibition of prostaglandin-synthesis on renal electrolyte excretion and concentrating ability in healthy man. *Prostaglandins Med*. 1978;1:341–9.

30. Vane JR, Botting RM. New insights into the mode of action of anti-inflammatory drugs. *Inflamm Res*. 1995;44:1–9.

31. Vane JR. Towards a better aspirin. *Nature*. 1994;367:215–6.

32. Frölich JC. A classification of NSAIDs according to the relative inhibition of cyclooxygenase isozymes. *Trends Pharmacol Sci*. 1997;18:30–4.

33. Rosenkranz B, Fischer C, Frölich JC. Effects of salicylic and acetylsalicylic acid alone and in combination on platelet aggregation and prostanoid synthesis in man. *Br J Clin Pharmacol*. 1986;21:309–17.

34. Stichtenoth DO, Wagner B, Frölich JC. Effects of meloxicam and indomethacin on cyclooxygenase pathways in healthy volunteers. *J Invest Med*. 1997;45:44–9.

35. Smith WL, Bell TG. Immunohistochemical localization of the prostaglandin forming cyclooxygenase in renal cortex. *Am J Physiol*. 1978;235:F451–F457.

36. O'Neill GP, Ford-Hutchinson AW. Expression of mRNA for cyclooxygenase-1 and -2 in human tissues. *FEBS Lett*. 1993;330:156–60.

37. Kömhoff M, Gröne H-J, Klein T, Seyberth HW, Nüsing RM. Localization of cyclooxygenase-1 and -2 in adult and fetal human kidney: implication for renal function. *Am J Physiol*. 1997;272:F460–F468.

38. Rosenkranz B, Náray-Fejes-Tóth A, Fejes-Tóth G, Fischer C, Sawada M, Frölich JC. Dexamethasone effect on prostanoid formation in healthy man. *Clin Sci*. 1985;68:681–5.

39. Frölich JC. Selectivity and meaningful classification of NSAIDs based on in vitro and in vivo analysis. *Trends Pharmacol Sci*. 1997;18:313.

40. Harris RC, McKanna JA, Akai Y, Jacobson HR, Dubois RN, Breyer MD. Cyclooxygenase-2 is associated with the macula densa of rat kidney and increases with salt restriction. *J Clin Invest*. 1994;94:2504–10.

41. Pairet M, Churchill L, Engelhardt G. Differential inhibition of cyclooxygenase 1 and 2 by NSAIDs. In: Bazan N, Botting J, Vane J, editors. *New Targets in Inflammation: Inhibitors of COX-2 or Adhesion Molecules*. London: Kluwer Academic Publishers and William Harvey Press; 1996:23–37.

42. Churchill L, Graham AC, Shih CK, Pauletti D, Farina PR, Grob PM. Selective inhibition of human cyclooxygenase-2 by meloxicam. *Inflammopharmacology*. 1996;4:125–35.

43. Bevis PJR, Bird HA, Lapham G. An open study to assess the safety and tolerability of meloxicam 15 mg in subjects with rheumatic disease and mild renal impairment. *Br J Rheumatol*. 1996;35(suppl 1):56–60.

44. Müller FO, Middle MV, Schall R, Terblanche J, Hundt HK, Groenewoud G. An evaluation of the interaction of meloxicam with frusemide in patients with compensated chronic cardiac failure. *Br J Clin Pharmacol.* 1997;44:393–8.

45. Degner F. Inhibition of COX-2 and its clinical relevance. Selective COX-2 inhibition, abstracts and posters, *19th ILAR Congress of Rheumatology, Singapore* 1997;31–5.

46. Stichtenoth DO, Wagner B, Frölich JC. Effect of selective inhibition of the inducible cyclooxygenase on renin release in healthy volunteers. *J Invest Med* 1998; in press.

47. Brunel P, Hornych A, Guyene TT, Sioufi A, Turri M, Menard J. Renal and endocrine effects of flosulide, after single and repeated administration to healthy volunteers. *Eur J Clin Pharmacol.* 1995;49:193–201.

Cyclooxygenase is expressed functionally in the renal thick ascending limb via angiotensin II stimulation of tumour necrosis factor-α

N. R. FERRERI, J. C. McGIFF AND C. P. VIO

The nephron is segmented relative to transport mechanisms, 12 or more segments having been identified, each segment having distinctive transport capabilities[1]. Less well appreciated is the uniqueness of each nephron segment with respect to arachidonic acid (AA) metabolism. Each nephron segment synthesizes a characteristic profile of eicosanoids that act as either modulators or mediators of the actions of hormones on tubular function[2,3]. Our initial studies on the rabbit medullary thick ascending limb (mTAL) of Henle's loop were directed towards examining the proposed modulatory action of prostaglandin E_2 (PGE_2) on ion movement in this segment occasioned by the study of Stokes on modulation by PGE_2 of chloride transport across the mTAL[4]. The mTAL, having a key role in the regulation of extracellular fluid volume, has on its contraluminal side a high concentration of the Na^+ pump (the Na^+–K^+-ATPase), a target of PGE_2 in the nephron[5].

AA METABOLISM BY THE NEPHRON

We isolated rabbit mTAL cells and, as a first step, characterized the principal AA products formed by the mTAL segment by adding [^{14}C]AA to a tubular suspension[6,7]. Radiolabelled arachidonate metabolites produced by the mTAL segregated into two principal peaks on reverse-phase HPLC; peak heights were not affected by indomethacin but were greatly diminished by inhibition of cytochrome P450 monooxygenase (CYP450). The principal CYP450-derived AA products synthesized by the rabbit mTAL were subsequently identified by gas chromatography–mass spectrometry as 19- and 20-hydroperoxyeicosatetra-enoates (HETEs), products of ω-1 and ω-hydroxylase activity, and 20-COOH HETE, a product of 20-HETE[2].

These studies indicated that the principal pathway of AA metabolism in the mTAL was via CYP450, designated as the third pathway of AA metabolism[8], and were interpreted as evidence that cyclooxygenase (COX), if it were present, was either a secondary pathway or one having negligible functional implications. Additional evidence supporting either a negligible or minor representation of COX in the mTAL was based on quantitative analysis of prostaglandin synthesis by radio- and enzyme-immunoassay of individual nephron segments[9]. This study, an analysis of segmental production of prostaglandins along the nephron, made several important points.

First, the principal COX product of the nephron is PGE_2, which exceeds formation of PGI_2 (measured as its hydrolysis product, 6-keto-$PGF_{1\alpha}$) and $PGF_{2\alpha}$ by 20-fold or more and thromboxane (TX) A_2 (measured as its hydrolysis product, TXB_2) by 100-fold.

Secondly, there is considerable variation in prostaglandin biosynthetic capacity amongst nephron segments, the proximal tubules and mTALs having the lowest or negligible capacity and the collecting tubules, the highest. These findings confirmed our study regarding the absence of detectable COX products in the rabbit mTAL, based on biochemical criteria, namely, on addition of AA to isolated mTAL cells transformation of AA proceeded exclusively via the CYP450 pathway[7].

Thirdly, there are notable quantitative differences between rat and rabbit relative to PGE_2 formation by the nephron, the rabbit showing 30- to 50-fold greater basal PGE_2 biosynthetic capacity. However, the PGE_2 profile along the nephron is similar for the rabbit and rat, collecting tubules showing high rates of PGE_2 synthesis and the proximal tubules and mTALs showing low or undetectable biosynthetic capabilities[9].

THE TAL SYNTHESIZES TUMOUR NECROSIS FACTOR-α

In addition to the evidence provided by quantitative microanalysis of segmental synthesis of prostaglandins along the nephron, indicating low or negligible ability to generate prostaglandins by the mTAL, an immunohistofluorescence procedure failed to detect COX in the mTAL[10], consistent with our findings. The initial study on localization of COX within the kidney by Smith and Wilkin on the renal medulla had detected the highest levels of COX antigenicity in the cells of the collecting tubules and lower levels in interstitial cells[11]. In a subsequent study on the immunohistochemical localization of COX in the renal cortex of the cow, guinea pig, rabbit, rat and sheep, COX antigenicity was detected in cortical collecting tubules and in the endothelial cells of renal arteries and arterioles of all mammals studied[10]. In contrast, COX antigenicity was absent in the TAL, a finding that, when viewed together with the evidence provided by biochemical and analytical criteria, had near absolute weight in eliminating a functionally significant prostaglandin (COX) representation in either cortical or medullary TALs.

The first challenge, and an unintentional one, to the seemingly impregnable bastion of 'the TAL without COX' was an outgrowth of our study on the functional consequences of a putative immunomodulator function of the mTAL[12]. Tumour necrosis factor (TNF)-α and interleukin-1 bind to the surface protein coating the mTAL, the Tamm–Horsfall glycoprotein, a cell-specific marker for the TAL to which an immunomodulatory function had been assigned by Hession et al.[13]. Isolated mTAL tubules from male rats were shown by Ferreri and colleagues[12] to express the gene for TNF-α and to release the cytokine in response to lipopolysaccharide (LPS). This study provided the incentive for linking changes in TNF-α production to altered ion transport in the mTAL. In view of the capacity of TNF-α to produce polyuria and natriuresis that were prevented by inhibition of COX[14] and the ability of TNF-α to induce COX-2 expression[15], we addressed a potential prostaglandin-dependent mechanism linking production of TNF-α to altered ion movement in the mTAL as reflected by changes in ^{86}Rb uptake, an index of epithelial cell transport[16].

Short-term incubation (<3 hours) of TNF-α with rat mTAL tubules did not affect ^{86}Rb uptake, whereas 24 hour exposure of tubules to TNF-α decreased ^{86}Rb uptake by more than 50%, an effect inhibited by indomethacin. Additional evidence for the involvement of a prostaglandin-dependent mechanism in the mTAL was uncovered on prolonged exposure (24 hour) of tubules to TNF-α; this resulted in increased PGE$_2$ production. Moreover, PGE$_2$ on short-term (30 minutes) incubation with mTAL tubules mimicked the effects of TNF-α by reducing ^{86}Rb uptake by isolated tubules[16].

This observation, when viewed together with the capacity of indomethacin to inhibit TNF-α modulation of ^{86}Rb uptake, constituted strong evidence that a prostaglandin, probably PGE$_2$, mediated the response of the mTAL to the cytokine (Figure 1). The initial observations were made on exogenous TNF-α which bypassed the potential contribution of endogenous TNF-α originating from mTAL cells. To determine the ability of endogenous TNF-α to modify ^{86}Rb uptake, we used LPS to stimulate TNF-α production in the mTAL. LPS inhibited ^{86}Rb uptake, an effect prevented by an anti-TNF-α antibody[16]. The time lag of upwards of four hours required for TNF-α to affect transport in the mTAL suggests that the TNF-α action was dependent on induction of COX-2 gene transcription followed by COX-2 protein expression in this segment, a point for which evidence has been recently obtained.

As angiotensin II (Ang II) affects ion transport in the TAL[17] and stimulates renal prostaglandin production[18], we next examined effects of Ang II on TAL transport via the mechanism involving TNF-α-dependent stimulation of PGE$_2$

Figure 1 Effect of TNF-α on ^{86}Rb uptake by TAL cells. Cells were pretreated for 24 hours with TNF-α alone (10[-9] M) (TNF), indomethacin(10[-6] M) and TNF-α (10[-9] M) (Indo + TNF), or SKF-525A (5×10[-5] M) and TNF-α (10[-9] M) (SKF + TNF). Experiments were run in pairs, with one group of cells incubated with vehicle and the other with a combination indicated above. Each bar represents mean±S.E. of five different cultures.

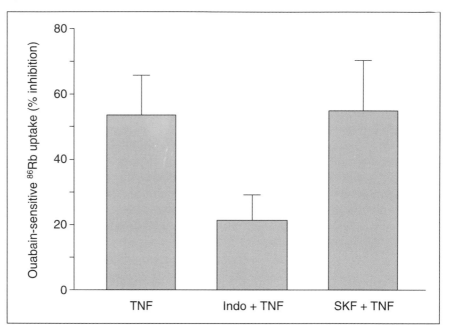

production[19]. Ang II (10[-11]–10[-7] M) on 3 hour exposure to TAL tubules increased TNF-α production several-fold, associated with a three-fold increase in TNF-α mRNA accumulation and comparable elevations in the concentration of PGE$_2$ in the incubate (Figure 2). An important distinction based on time-dependent effects of Ang II on ^{86}Rb uptake by the TAL was observed, viz. a PGE$_2$-dependent mechanism was involved in the long term (three hour) and a CYP450 (20-HETE)-dependent mechanism in the short-term (15 minutes) effects of Ang II on ion movement in the TAL[19].

THE mTAL EXPRESSES COX-2 CONSTITUTIVELY

While the functional studies on a COX-dependent mechanism initiated by TNF-α in the mTAL were in progress, a morphological study on the localization of COX-2 to the rat TAL and macula densa was published[20]. Chronic dietary salt depletion (14 days) produced a three-fold increase in COX-2 immunoreactivity in cells thought to be macula densa cells as well as those of the adjacent TAL. The macula densa is an extension of the TAL and is the renal tubular component of the juxtaglomerular apparatus that includes the glomerular afferent artery and

Figure 2 Angiotensin II (Ang II) increases PGE$_2$ production. TAL tubules were incubated with the indicated doses of Ang II for 3 hours at 37°C. At the end of the incubation period, PGE$_2$ levels in cell-free supernatants were determined by an enzyme-linked immunosorbent assay. Data are means±S.D. *P<0.005, n=3.

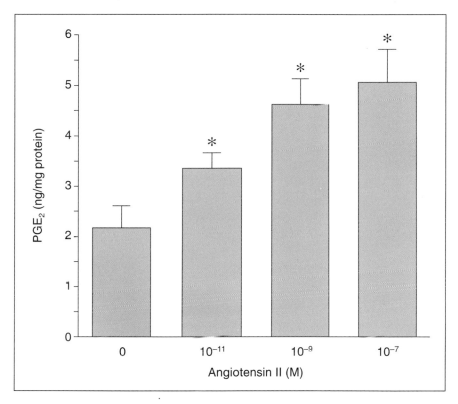

contiguous mesangium. The macula densa acts 'as both sensor and effector of total salt and volume homeostasis'[21]. The functional implications, therefore, of this study on localization of a constitutive COX-2 to the macula densa are great as the macula densa is a key component in tubulo–glomerular feedback, the mechanism that governs the regulation of extracellular fluid volume by determining delivery of solute to the nephron.

However, two recent studies, while confirming localization of COX-2 to the TAL, have not identified COX-2 in the macula densa although confusion could well have arisen regarding localization of COX-2 positive cells to the macula densa because of the proximity to the glomerulus of COX-2 positive cells in the TAL[22,23]. The latter were distinguished from the cells of the macula densa as TAL cells demonstrate Tamm–Horsfall protein, a specific marker of the TAL, which is absent from the macula densa[22]. Thus, a subset of COX-2 positive cells were unequivocally identified as belonging to the TAL because of co-localization of Tamm–Horsfall protein. Moreover, COX-2 staining of TAL cells was not abolished by treatment with glucocorticoids, suggesting the constitutive character of COX-2 in the TAL segment of the rat nephron[22]. COX-2 antigenicity was not observed in other segments of the rat nephron nor in glomeruli, nor in vascular and interstitial cells. As COX-2 is expressed at low levels in the rat kidney, based on an RNA sample of the whole organ, localization of COX-2 to scattered TAL cells indicates 'a high message in a small subpopulation of cells'[22]. Although only a small number of TAL cells express COX-2, this finding, nonetheless, has important physiological implications for the cells that demonstrate detectable COX-2. As low salt intake increased the number of TAL cells expressing COX-2[20], involvement of the renin–angiotensin system, in particular an Ang II-mediated effect on the mTAL, is implicated. We found that Ang II stimulated prostaglandin production by the TAL via a TNF-α-dependent mechanism that mediated alterations in ion transport in the mTAL[19]. Further, Ang II increased TNF-α mRNA and TNF-α release from the mTAL associated with expression of COX-2. A caveat regarding the important challenges to the localization of COX-2 to the macula densa[20], namely salt depletion, may be a necessary condition for expressing COX-2 in the macula densa.

It is at the mTAL that the interactions of Ang II, TNF-α and COX-2 have the greatest functional implications for regulating salt and water excretion and body fluid homeostasis. These interrelationships involving vasoactive hormones, cytokines and COX have been magnified by an in vivo study of Ang II-dependent hypertension[24]. Infusion of Ang II to rats for 10 days resulted in hypertension that was exacerbated by administration of anti-TNF-α antiserum which neutralized the activity of soluble and membrane-bound TNF-α, suggesting that TNF-α is an essential component of an antihypertensive mechanism that opposes the pressor response to Ang II. Moreover, mTAL tubules isolated from rats made hypertensive with Ang II infused for 10 days showed several-fold greater production of both TNF-α and PGE_2 than mTAL tubules obtained from normotensive rats, suggesting that TNF-α and PGE_2 act in concert to counterregulate the activity of pressor hormones (Figures 3 and 4).

COX-1 AND COX-2 AFFECT RENAL DIFFERENTIATION AND MATURATION

The functional significance of renal COX-2 was highlighted in mice in which the neuronal nitric oxide synthase (nNOS) gene was disrupted (nNOS-/-)[25]. Although renal renin content was reduced under basal conditions in nNOS knockout mice, renin increase in response to a low sodium diet was unimpaired. NS-398, the selective inhibitor of COX-2, however, blocked the elevation in renal renin content evoked by dietary sodium restriction. This study eliminated an NO-linked increase in prostaglandin production involving nNOS (but not iNOS/cNOS) as an essential component in the mechanism that elevated renal renin production when challenged by low sodium intake. Moreover, a product of COX-2 is essential to this demonstration.

Figure 3 Effects of infusion of angiotensin II (Ang II) on production of TNF-α by mTAL tubules. Tubules were isolated from rats that had been infused with Ang II or vehicle and incubated for three hours at 37°C. Production of TNF-α was measured by an enzyme-linked immunosorbent assay. The data are the means of duplicate assay determinations; the S.D.s were less than 5% in all cases.

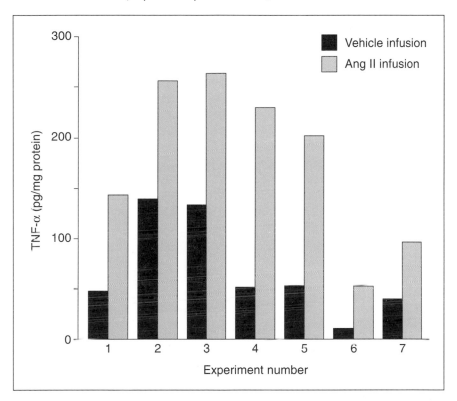

The foetal kidney is a rich source of prostaglandins, synthesized primarily by COX-2, that are involved in the rat 'in the maturation of individual nephrons rather than in global physiological phenomena'[23]. Two parallel lines of evidence, each based on suppressing prostaglandin production in mammalian foetuses, arrive at the same general conclusion; namely, foetal renal prostaglandins, particularly PGE_2, are required for growth and differentiation of the kidney. The first line of evidence was provided by targeted disruption of COX-2 in mice[26,27]. In contrast to COX-1 knockout mice[28], COX-2 knockout mice demonstrated small kidneys with few functional nephrons, exhibiting immature glomeruli and manifest impairment of postnatal nephrogenesis (in rodents maturation of nephrons continues through the first two postnatal weeks). These mice die of uraemia within three to four months. Chronic administration of non-steroidal anti-inflammatory drugs (NSAIDs) to pregnant Rhesus monkeys reproduced many of the features described in COX-2 knockout mice[29]. Similar renal lesions have been reported in infants who died postnatally, and whose mothers gave a history of

Figure 4 Effects of infusion of angiotensin II (Ang II) on production of PGE_2 by mTAL tubules. Tubules were isolated from rats that had been infused with Ang II or vehicle and incubated for three hours at 37°C. PGE_2 content in the cell-free supernatants was determined by an enzyme-linked immunosorbent assay. The data are the means of duplicate assay determinations; the S.D.s were less than 5% in all cases.

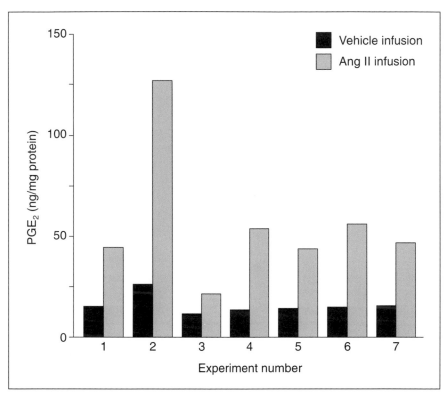

chronic ingestion of COX inhibitors during pregnancy[30]. In foetuses exposed to NSAIDs, even late in pregnancy, renal abnormalities have been described; foetal lambs demonstrated decreased renal blood flow and disturbances in regulating salt and water excretion when administered indomethacin late in gestation[31].

Zhang et al.[23] have studied systematically the expression of COX-2 in the rat kidney and have linked COX-2 to the differentiation and maturation of nephrons. Based on Northern and Western analysis, expression of COX-2 mRNA and protein, respectively, became discernible by the 16th embryonic day, remaining low until birth, peaking in the first two postnatal weeks, and then, subsiding to the low levels characteristic of adults by about the sixth week postnatally. An interesting negative correlation of glucocorticoids with changing expression of renal COX-2 emerged when examining changes in glucocorticoid levels in rodents during the postnatal period, in view of the ability of glucocorticoids to inhibit expression of COX-2[32]. Increased expression of renal COX-2 occurred at a time, the first two to three postnatal weeks, when plasma levels of glucocorticoids were very low[33] suggesting derepression of COX-2. As noted previously, despite the very low levels of COX-2 mRNA and immunoreactive protein in adult rats, a subset of TAL cells continue to express COX-2 message and protein through the adult period[23].

As indicated by the immunocytochemistry studies of Smith and Bell[10], species differences were evident in localizing COX to specific structures. The study of Kömhoff et al. emphasizes the differences between human and rat kidneys[34]. In the adult human whole kidney, COX-1 and COX-2 mRNA levels were expressed basally almost equally in the medulla, confirming the findings of O'Neill and Ford-Hutchinson[35]. COX-1 immunoreactive protein in the adult was present in glomeruli, vasculature and interstitial cells and in the collecting ducts and thin loop of Henle of the nephron[34]. An important finding in the adult human kidney was the prominent localization of COX-2 to both endothelial and smooth muscle cells of the vasculature and to a specific structure of the glomerulus, the podocyte, a contractile element of the glomerulus, suggesting involvement of products of COX-2 in the regulation of glomerular perfusion and filtration[34]. These findings raise the question as to whether a selective COX-2 inhibitor would be sufficiently renal sparing in man so as to warrant its use in the treatment of patients with diseases requiring long-term therapy with NSAIDs such as rheumatoid arthritis. A recent clinical study on flosulide, a selective COX-2 inhibitor, suggested that the therapeutic objective of treating a disease with a COX-2 selective NSAID, while preserving renal function, may not be realizable[36].

Acknowledgements

This work was supported by NIH grants HL34300 and R01-25394 (JCM), American Heart Association grant 9740001N and R01HL56423 (NRF), and by Fondo Nacional de Desarrollo Científico y Tecnológico (Fondecyt, Chile) grant 1980951 (CPV). Dr Ferreri is an Established Investigator of the American Heart Association. The authors thank Ms Gail D. Price for assistance in the preparation of this manuscript.

REFERENCES

1. Knepper M, Burg M. Organization of nephron function. *Am J Physiol.* 1983;244:F579–F589.
2. Carroll MA, Sala A, Dunn CE, McGiff JC, Murphy RC. Structural identification of cytochrome P450-dependent arachidonate metabolites formed by rabbit medullary thick ascending limb cells. *J Biol Chem.* 1991;266:12306–12.
3. Omata K, Ibraham NG, Schwartzman ML. Renal cytochrome P-450-arachidonic acid metabolism: localization and hormonal regulation in SHR. *Am J Physiol.* 1992;262:F591–F599.
4. Stokes JB. Effect of prostaglandin E$_2$ on chloride transport across the rabbit thick ascending limb of Henle. *J Clin Invest.* 1979;61:495–502.

5. Wald H, Scherzer P, Rubinger D, Popovtzer MM. Effect of indomethacin in vivo and PGE$_2$ in vitro on mTAL Na-K-ATPase of the rat kidney. *Pflügers Arch.* 1990;415:648–50.

6. Ferreri NR, Schwartzman M, Ibraham NG, Chander PN, McGiff JC. Arachidonic acid metabolism in a cell suspension isolated from rabbit renal outer medulla. *J Pharmacol Exp Ther.* 1984;231:441–8.

7. Schwartzman M, Ferreri NR, Carroll MA, Songu-Mize E, McGiff JC. Renal cytochrome P450-related arachidonate metabolite inhibits (Na$^+$-K$^+$)ATPase. *Nature.* 1985;314:620–2.

8. Schwartzman M, Carroll MA, Ibraham NG, Ferreri NR, Songu-Mize E, McGiff JC. Renal arachidonic acid metabolism. The third pathway. *Hypertension.* 1985;7(suppl I): I136–I144.

9. Bonvalet J-P, Pradelles P, Farman N. Segmental synthesis and actions of prostaglandins along the nephron. *Am J Physiol.* 1987;253:F377–F387.

10. Smith WL, Bell TG. Immunohistochemical localization of the prostaglandin-forming cyclooxygenase in renal cortex. *Am J Physiol.* 1978;235:F451–F457.

11. Smith WL, Wilkin GP. Immunochemistry of prostaglandin endoperoxide-forming cyclooxygenases: the detection of the cyclooxygenases in rat, rabbit and guinea pig kidneys by immunofluoresence. *Prostaglandins.* 1977;13:873–92.

12. Macica CM, Escalante BA, Conners MS, Ferreri NR. TNF production by the medullary thick ascending limb of Henle's loop. *Kidney Int.* 1994;46:113–21.

13. Hession C, Decker JM, Sherblom AP, Kumar S, Yue CC, Mattaliano RJ et al. A renal ligand for lymphokines. *Science.* 1987;237:1479–84.

14. Van-Lanschot JJ, Mealy K, Jacobs DO, Evan DO, Wilmore DW. Splenectomy attenuates the inappropriate diuresis associated with tumor necrosis factor administration. *Surg Gynecol Obstet.* 1991;172:293–7.

15. Yamamoto K, Arakawa T, Ueda N, Yamamoto S. Transcriptional roles of nuclear factor κB and nuclear factor-interleukin-6 in the tumor necrosis factor α-dependent induction of cyclooxygenase-2 in MC3T3-E1 cells. *J Biol Chem.* 1995;270:31315–20.

16. Escalante BA, Ferreri NR, Dunn CE, McGiff JC. Cytokines affect ion transport in primary cultured thick ascending limb of Henle's loop cells. *Am J Physiol.* 1994;266:C1568–C1576.

17. Capasso G, Unwin R, Ciani F, De-Santo NG, DeTommaso G, Russo F et al. Bicarbonate transport along the loop of Henle. II. Effects of acid-base, dietary, and neurohumoral determinants. *J Clin Invest.* 1994;94:830–8.

18. McGiff JC, Crowshaw K, Terragno NA, Lonigro AJ. Renal prostaglandins: possible regulators of the renal actions of pressor hormone. *Nature.* 1970;227:1255–7.

19. Ferreri NR, Escalante BA, Zhao Y, An S-J, McGiff JC. Angiotensin II induces TNF production by the thick ascending limb: functional implications. *Am J Physiol.* 1998;274:F148–F155.

20. Harris RC, McKanna JA, Akai Y, Jacobson HR, Dubois RN, Breyer MD. Cyclooxygenase-2 is associated with the macula densa of rat kidney and increases with salt restriction. *J Clin Invest.* 1994;94:2504–10.

21. Harris RC. The macula densa: recent developments. *J Hypertension.* 1996;14:815–22.

22. Vio CP, Cespedes C, Gallardo P, Masferrer JL. Renal identification of cyclooxygenase-2 in a subset of thick ascending limb cells. *Hypertension.* 1997;30:687–92.

23. Zhang M-Z, Wang J-L, Cheng H-F, Harris RC, McKanna JA. Cyclooxygenase-2 in rat nephron development. *Am J Physiol.* 1997;273:F994–F1002.

24. Ferreri NR, Zhao Y, Takizawa H, McGiff JC. Tumor necrosis factor-α-angiotensin inter-actions and regulation of blood pressure. *J Hypertension.* 1997;15:1481–4.

25. Harding P, Sigmon DH, Alfie ME, Huang PL, Fishman MC, Beierwaltes WH, Carretero OA. Cyclooxygenase-2 mediates increased renal renin content induced by low-sodium diet. *Hypertension.* 1997;29:297–302.

26. Morham SG, Lagenbach R, Loftin CD, Tiano HF, Vouloumanos N, Jennette JC et al. Prostaglandin synthase 2 gene disruption causes severe renal pathologies in the mouse. *Cell*. 1995;83:473–82.

27. Dinchuk JE, Car BD, Focht RJ, Johnston JJ, Jaffee BD, Covington MB et al. Renal abnormalities and an altered inflammatory response in mice lacking cyclooxygenase II. *Nature*. 1995;378:406–9.

28. Langenbach R, Morham SG, Tiano HF, Loftin CD, Ghanayem BI, Chulada PC et al. Prostaglandin synthase 1 gene disruption in mice reduced arachidonic acid-induced inflammation and indomethacin-induced gastric ulceration. *Cell*. 1995;83:483–92.

29. Novy MJ. Effects of indomethacin on labor, fetal oxygenation, and fetal development in rhesus monkeys. *Adv Prostaglandin Thromboxane Leukot Res*. 1978;4:285–300.

30. Van Der Heijden BJ, Carlus C, Narcy F, Bavoux F, Delezoide AL, Gubler MC. Persistent anuria, neonatal death, and renal microcystic lesions after prenatal exposure to indomethacin. *Am J Obstet Gynecol*. 1994;171:617–23.

31. Matson JR, Stokes JB, Robillard JE. Effects of inhibition of prostaglandin synthesis on fetal renal function. *Kidney Int*. 1981;20:621–7.

32. Masferrer JL, Seibert K, Zweifel B, Needleman P. Endogenous glucocorticoids regulate an inducible cyclooxygenase enzyme. *Proc Natl Acad Sci USA*. 1992;89:3917–21.

33. Henning SJ. Plasma concentrations of total and free corticosterone during development in the rat. *Am J Physiol*. 1978;235:E451–E456.

34. Kömhoff M, Gröne H-J, Klein T, Seyberth HW, Nüsing RM. Localization of cyclooxygenase-1 and -2 in adult and fetal human kidney: implication for renal function. *Am J Physiol*. 1997;272:F460–F468.

35. O'Neill GP, Ford-Hutchinson AW. Expression of mRNA for cyclooxygenase-1 and cyclooxygenase-2 in human tissues. *FEBS Lett*. 1993;330:156–60.

36. Emery P. Pharmacology, safety data and therapeutics of COX-2 inhibitors. In: Vane J, Botting J, Botting R, editors. *Improved Non-Steroid Anti-Inflammatory Drugs*. London: Kluwer Academic Publishers and William Harvey Press; 1996:229–42.

Expression of cyclooxygenase-2 in human gastric carcinoma

A. RISTIMÄKI

Gastric cancer is one of the most common and lethal malignancies in the world[1]. The prognosis for this disease is poor, since the late appearance of the symptoms delays the patient from seeking medical treatment. At present the only successful treatment is early diagnosis and total removal of the tumour by surgery. However, early detection of stomach cancer is difficult, and in most western countries the 5 year survival rate is less than 20%[2]. Although stomach cancer is characterized by multiple gene changes, such as those of oncogenes, tumour suppressor genes, cell cycle regulators, cell–cell adhesion molecules, and growth factors or their receptors[3], the pathogenesis of this disease is still not completely understood.

More than 90% of stomach cancers are adenocarcinomas, which are divided into intestinal and diffuse types by the Laurén classification[4]. Interestingly, the pattern of genetic changes differs depending on the histological typing of the gastric cancer[3]. Thus, the intestinal and diffuse gastric tumours may have different genetic backgrounds. Further, while the diffuse type lacks well-recognized precursor changes, the intestinal type is preceded by a sequence of events, such as chronic atrophic gastritis, intestinal metaplasia, dysplasia, intramucosal carcinoma, and finally invasive cancer[5]. However, while atrophic gastritis and intestinal metaplasia are associated with intestinal gastric tumours in retrospective studies, only epithelial dysplasia has a predictive value for this malignancy[5].

USE OF NSAIDS REDUCES THE RISK OF GASTROINTESTINAL CARCINOMAS

Record linkage studies in Finland and Sweden have found a lower incidence of gastrointestinal cancer, including gastric cancer, among patients with rheumatoid arthritis than in the general population[6–8]. Since these patients use aspirin and other nonsteroidal anti-inflammatory drugs (NSAIDs) in high doses for prolonged periods of time, it is possible that these drugs are responsible for the reduction in the cancer incidence. In addition, a large prospective mortality study found that the use of aspirin is associated with reduced risk of oesophageal, gastric, and colorectal cancers[9]. These results have now been confirmed in several studies for the colorectal cancer (reviewed in reference 10) and by a recent study for the cancer of the oesophagus and the stomach[11].

COX-2 IS THE ONLY KNOWN TARGET FOR THE CHEMOPREVENTIVE EFFECT OF NSAIDS

The best known target of NSAIDs is cyclooxygenase (COX), the rate-limiting enzyme in the conversion of arachidonic acid to prostanoids[12]. Two COX genes have been cloned (COX-1 and COX-2), and these share over 60% identity at the amino acid level and have similar enzymatic activities[12–14]. The most striking difference between the COX genes is in the regulation of their expression. While COX-1 is constitutively expressed, and the expression is not usually regulated, expression of COX-2 is low or not detectable under basal conditions, and it is highly induced in response to cell activation by hormones, tumour promoters, growth factors, and pro-inflammatory agents. Thus, COX-1 is considered to be a housekeeping gene, and prostanoids synthesized via the COX-1 pathway are thought to be responsible for cytoprotection of the stomach, for vasodilatation in the kidney, and for production of a pro-aggregatory prostanoid, thromboxane, by platelets. In contrast, COX-2 is an inducible, immediate-early gene, and its pathophysiological role is involved with inflammation, reproduction, and carcinogenesis.

Recent studies suggest that COX-2 is associated with colon carcinogenesis and that it is one of the targets for the chemopreventive effect of NSAIDs. First, elevated levels of COX-2 mRNA and protein, but not those of COX-1, were found in human colon carcinomas[15–17]. Second, expression of COX-2 is elevated in carcinogen-induced rat colonic tumours[18] and in the *Min* mouse adenoma, which is a model for familial adenomatous polyposis (FAP)[19,20]. Further, four different selective COX-2 inhibitors suppress adenoma formation or chemically-induced aberrant crypt foci in the rodent gastrointestinal tract[21–24]. Finally, genetic disruption of COX-2 suppresses polyp formation in $Apc^{\Delta 716}$-knockout mice (reference 24 and chapter by Dr Taketo in this volume). However, one should bear in mind that COX-2 may not be the sole target even for so-called COX-2 selective drugs[25], and that only clinical trials will show whether COX-2 selective drugs prove to be beneficial in the prevention and/or treatment of gastrointestinal cancers.

COX-2 EXPRESSION IS ELEVATED IN GASTRIC CARCINOMA

Normal gastrointestinal tissues contain almost exclusively the COX-1 isoform[26]. Some COX-2 mRNA may be detected with more sensitive methods than the traditional Northern blot hybridization assay of total RNA[27,28], but no COX-2 protein has been found in healthy stomach tissue[26,28-30]. However, the opposite pattern of expression of COX isoforms may be found in gastrointestinal diseases, since COX-2 mRNA and protein are elevated in chemically-induced gastric ulcers and bowel inflammation in rodents[30,31]. Interestingly, inhibition of COX-2 delayed healing of gastric lesions and exacerbated colonic injury in these experimental models[30,31]. Thus, although selective COX-2 inhibitors spare normal gastrointestinal prostanoid synthesis, and therefore do not promote gastric injury, they may interfere with wound healing and resistance to inflammation-induced injury.

We reported recently that human gastric adenocarcinoma tissues contain significantly higher levels of COX-2 mRNA than their paired mucosal specimens devoid of cancer cells[28] (Figure 1a). In contrast, COX-1 mRNA levels were not elevated in the carcinoma (Figure 1b). An identical pattern of COX expression was recently reported in human stomach tumours, when Soydan et al. detected

Figure 1 Expression of COX-2 mRNA is elevated in gastric carcinoma. (a) Ratio of COX-2 mRNA to GAPDH mRNA. (b) Ratio of COX-1 mRNA to GAPDH mRNA. Total RNA was extracted from 10 gastric carcinoma specimens and from their paired controls (from antrum and corpus) that contained no cancer cells and analysed using Northern blot hybridization. Hybridization was performed with probes for human COX-1 and COX-2 and with glyceraldehyde-3-phosphate dehydrogenase (GAPDH) as the loading control. Values (means±S.E.M.) in the graphs represent the ratio of COX mRNAs to GAPDH mRNA calculated from the arbitrary densitometric units, which indicate that gastric carcinoma tissues expressed significantly higher levels of COX-2 mRNA than did the control samples (P<0.05). COX-1 mRNA levels were not elevated in the carcinoma tissues. Note that the three carcinomas that expressed the lowest levels of COX-2 were at or below the detection limit of the Northern blot assay. These samples were further analysed with reverse transcriptase–polymerase chain reaction, and two of the three carcinoma specimens were found to contain elevated COX-2 mRNA levels when compared to their respective controls (see reference 28).

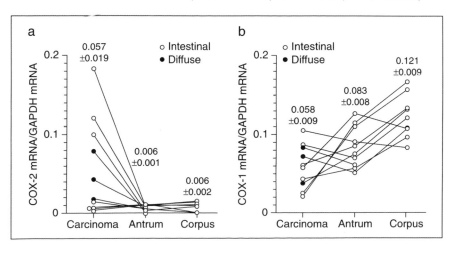

COX proteins by using Western blotting[29]. In our studies, the most intense COX-2 protein staining is localized in cancer cells (Figure 2), which is consistent with data obtained from human colon carcinoma tissues[17].

Elevated expression of COX-2 mRNA was not limited to the intestinal type of gastric cancer, since each of the three diffuse carcinomas analysed contained higher levels of the COX-2 transcript than their respective controls (Figure 1a). However, our recent unpublished data indicate that while the great majority of the intestinal type carcinomas are positive for the COX-2 protein, it is a rare event to find a positive diffuse type carcinoma when using immunohistochemistry. This apparent discrepancy may be due to deficiency of translation of COX-2 in the diffuse type carcinomas or to expression of COX-2 at sites other than the neoplastic cells themselves. Interestingly, we found positive COX-2 immunostaining in stromal cells (fibroblasts, mononuclear leukocytes and vascular endothelium) at sites of ulcerations that are frequently associated with this disease. Since normal colonic epithelium expresses only low levels of COX-2 mRNA and elevated levels are found in over 40% of premalignant colonic adenomas and in almost 90% of colon carcinomas[15], it is possible that such a gradient of gene expression is also found in the stomach. Our unpublished data also indicate that COX-2 is expressed in dysplasias of the stomach. All this suggests that COX-2 protein expression is mainly associated with the intestinal type of gastric carcinoma and with the pre-malignant lesions leading to it.

MECHANISM AND SIGNIFICANCE OF COX-2 OVEREXPRESSION IN CARCINOGENESIS

Initiation of carcinogenesis is dependent on malignant transformation. Overexpression of either COX-2[32] or COX-1[33] does not transform cells.

Figure 2 Immunostaining for COX-2 in gastric carcinoma tissues. (a) Immunohistological staining for COX-2 showed cytoplasmic staining (red-brown colour) in the cancer cells (black arrows), but not in the surrounding stroma (white arrows). An IgG fraction of polyclonal murine COX-2 antiserum (Cayman Chemicals, Ann Arbor, MI, USA) was used as the primary antibody. (b) When normal rabbit IgG was used as the primary antibody, tissue sections showed no staining.

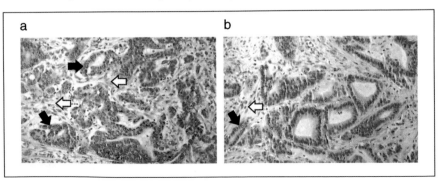

However, several lines of evidence indicate that expression of COX-2 is induced in response to cellular transformation. First, COX-2 cDNA was originally identified from chicken embryo fibroblasts transformed with v-*src*, which is an oncogene from the Rous sarcoma virus[34]. Second, transformation of rat intestinal epithelial (RIE) cells with H-*ras* oncogene[32] and of mammary epithelial cells with either *src* or *ras*[35] induced COX-2 expression. Further, *src*-induced COX-2 expression was downregulated by dominant negative *ras*[35]. In addition to oncogenes, COX-2 may also be induced by inactivation of anti-oncogenes, as has been shown in adenomas of *Min* mice[19,20] and of *Apc*[Δ716]-knockout mice[24]. The mechanism behind transformation-induced COX-2 expression is associated with increased transcription[35]. However, since COX-2 mRNA is very unstable and its stability can be modulated[36,37], one should not exclude the possibility of regulation at the post-transcriptional level. Thus, it seems clear that COX-2 overexpression is not sufficient for malignant transformation, but that malignant transformation is an important mechanism in induction of constitutive COX-2 expression.

Tumour formation is dependent on clonal expansion due to increased growth and/or reduced death. A COX-2 selective compound, SC-58125, inhibited the growth of the H-*ras*-transformed RIE cells via inhibition of cell proliferation and by induction of apoptosis, but it had no effect on growth of control cells[32]. The same group has also reported that SC-58125 inhibits tumour formation in nude mice by the HCA-7 human colon carcinoma cell line that expresses high levels of COX-2, but tumours formed by the HCT-116 cell line that lacks COX-2 were not inhibited[38]. Similarly, another COX-2 specific inhibitor, NS-398, suppressed proliferation of a gastric carcinoma cell line (MKN45) that expresses high steady-state levels of COX-2 mRNA, but was without effect in cell lines (MKN28 and KATO III) that express low levels of COX-2 mRNA[39]. Further, stable transfection of the RIE cells with COX-2 alters both their rate of programmed cell death and their adhesion to the extracellular matrix[40]. Finally, SC-58125 induced apoptosis in HCA-7 cells that was inhibited by prostaglandin (PG) E_2, which effect may depend on induction of Bcl-2 expression[41]. Interestingly, in a mouse skin cancer model, the antitumour effect of indomethacin was reversed by $PGF_{2\alpha}$ but not by PGE_2[42]. This may indicate that a different pattern of prostanoid receptors operates in different epithelial cell compartments. All this indicates that overexpression of COX-2 may promote proliferation of transformed epithelial cells by protecting them from apoptosis. Whether these properties are dependent on prostanoids needs further investigation.

Also, prostanoids may promote tumour progression by inducing proteinase production, and thus tumour invasion and metastasis[43], and by stimulating angiogenesis, the sprouting of capillaries from pre-existing blood vessels[33,44]. In fact, we have shown that although stable transfection of COX-1 does not stimulate growth or reduce apoptosis of immortalized ECV endothelial cells in vitro, only the COX-1-overexpressing cells form tumours in nude mice in vivo[33]. Tumours formed by COX-1-transfected cells contained numerous host-derived vessels, which indicates induction of angiogenesis. One possible explanation for COX-induced angiogenesis is elevated production of PGE_2, which has been shown to stimulate synthesis of an important angiogenic factor, vascular endothelial growth factor, probably via the EP_2 receptor[45,46]. Interestingly, basic fibroblast growth factor and epidermal growth factor induced COX-2 expression in the rat sponge implant model and the angiogenic response induced by these polypeptide growth factors was suppressed by indomethacin and by the COX-2 selective inhibitor NS-398[47]. All this suggests that COX-2 may be up-regulated in tumour cells by growth factors derived from the cancer cells themselves, or from stromal cells, and that the COX-2-derived prostanoids may modulate production of angiogenic factors and proteases, which would then lead to more aggressive growth and invasion.

Acknowledgements

Supported by the Academy of Finland and Helsinki University Central Hospital Research Funds.

REFERENCES

1. Coleman MP, Esteve J, Damiecki P, Arslan A, Renard H. In: Trends in Cancer Incidence and Mortality. Lyon: *IARC Scientific Publications No. 121*; 1993:193–224.
2. Wanebo HJ, Kennedy BJ, Chmiel J, Steele GJ, Winchester D, Osteen R. Cancer of the stomach. A patient care study by the American College of Surgeons. *Ann Surg.* 1993;218:583–92.
3. Tahara E, Semba S, Tahara H. Molecular biological observations in gastric cancer. *Semin Oncol.* 1996;23:307–15.
4. Laurén P. The two histological main types of gastric carcinoma: diffuse and so-called intestinal-type carcinomas: an attempt at a histo-clinical classification. *Acta Path Microbiol Scand.* 1965;64:31–49.
5. Antonioli DA. Precursors of gastric carcinoma: a critical review with a brief description of early (curable) gastric cancer. *Hum Pathol.* 1994;25:994–1005.
6. Isomäki HA, Hakulinen T, Joutsenlahti U. Excess risk of lymphomas, leukemia, and myeloma in patients with rheumatoid arthritis. *J Chron Dis.* 1978;31:691–6.
7. Laakso M, Mutru O, Isomäki H, Koota K. Cancer mortality in patients with rheumatoid arthritis. *J Rheumatol.* 1986;13:522–6.
8. Gridley G, McLaughlin JK, Ekbom A, Klareskog L, Adami H-O, Hacker DG et al. Incidence of cancer among patients with rheumatoid arthritis. *J Natl Cancer Inst.* 1993;85:307–11.
9. Thun MJ, Namboodiri MM, Calle EE, Flanders WD, Heath Jr CW. Aspirin use and risk of fatal cancer. *Cancer Res.* 1993;53:1322–7.
10. Giardiello FM, Offerhaus GJA, DuBois RN. The role of nonsteroidal anti-inflammatory drugs in colorectal cancer prevention. *Eur J Cancer.* 1995;31A:1071–6.
11. Farrow DC, Vaughan TL, Hansten PD, Stanford JL, Risch HA, Gammon MD et al. Use of aspirin and other nonsteroidal anti-inflammatory drugs and risk of esophageal and gastric cancer. *Cancer Epidemiol Biomark Prev.* 1998;7:97–102.
12. Vane JR, Botting RM. Mechanism of action of aspirin-like drugs. *Semin Arthritis Rheum.* 1997;26:2–10.

13. Smith WL, Garavito RM, DeWitt DL. Prostaglandin endoperoxide H synthases (cyclooxygenases)-1 and -2. *J Biol Chem.* 1996;271:33157–60.
14. Williams CS, DuBois RN. Prostaglandin endoperoxide synthase: Why two isoforms? *Am J Physiol.* 1996;270:G393–G400.
15. Eberhart CE, Coffey RJ, Radhika A, Giardiello FM, Ferrenbach S, DuBois RN. Up-regulation of cyclooxygenase 2 gene expression in human colorectal adenomas and adenocarcinomas. *Gastroenterology.* 1994;107:1183–8.
16. Kargman SL, O'Neill GP, Vickers PJ, Evans JF, Mancini JA, Jothy S. Expression of prostaglandin G/H synthase-1 and -2 protein in human colon cancer. *Cancer Res.* 1995;55:2556–9.
17. Sano H, Kawahito Y, Wilder RL, Hashiramoto A, Mukai S, Asai K et al. Expression of cyclooxygenase-1 and -2 in human colorectal cancer. *Cancer Res.* 1995;55:3785- 9.
18. DuBois RN, Radhika A, Reddy BS, Entingh AJ. Increased cyclooxygenase-2 levels in carcinogen-induced rat colonic tumors. *Gastroenterology.* 1996;110:1259–62.
19. Boolbol SK, Dannenberg AJ, Chadburn A, Martucci C, Guo X, Ramonetti JT et al. Cyclooxygenase-2 overexpression and tumor formation are blocked by sulindac in a murine model of familial adenomatous polyposis. *Cancer Res.* 1996;56:2556–60.
20. Williams CS, Luongo C, Radhika A, Zhang T, Lamps LW, Nanney LB et al. Elevated cyclooxygenase-2 levels in *Min* mouse adenomas. *Gastroenterology.* 1996;111:1134–40.
21. Takahashi M, Fukutake M, Yokota S, Ishida K, Wakabayashi K, Sugimura T. Suppression of azoxymethane-induced aberrant crypt foci in rat colon by nimesulide, a selective inhibitor of cyclooxygenase 2. *J Cancer Res Clin Oncol.* 1996;122:219–22.
22. Reddy BS, Rao CV, Seibert K. Evaluation of cyclooxygenase-2 inhibitor for potential chemopreventive properties in colon carcinogenesis. *Cancer Res.* 1996;56:4566–9.
23. Yoshimi N, Kawabata K, Hara A, Matsunaga K, Yamada Y, Mori H. Inhibitory effect of NS-398, a selective cyclooxygenase-2 inhibitor, on azoxymethane-induced aberrant crypt foci in colon carcinogenesis of F344 rats. *Jpn J Cancer Res.* 1997;88:1044–51.
24. Oshima M, Dinchuk JE, Kargman SL, Oshima H, Hancock B, Kwong E et al. Suppression of intestinal polyposis in *Apc*$^{\Delta/16}$ knockout mice by inhibition of cyclooxygenase 2 (COX-2). *Cell.* 1996;87:803–9.
25. Elder DJE, Halton DE, Hague A, Paraskeva C. Induction of apoptotic cell death in human colorectal carcinoma cell lines by a cyclooxygenase-2 (COX-2)-selective nonsteroidal anti-inflammatory drug: independence from COX-2 protein expression. *Clin Cancer Res.* 1997;3:1679–83.
26. Kargman S, Charleson S, Cartwright M, Frank J, Riendeau D, Mancini J et al. Characterization of prostaglandin G/H synthase 1 and 2 in rat, dog, monkey, and human gastrointestinal tracts. *Gastroenterology.* 1996;111:445–54.
27. O'Neill GP, Ford-Hutchinson AW. Expression of mRNA for cyclooxygenase-1 and cyclooxygenase-2 in human tissues. *FEBS Lett.* 1993;330:156–60.
28. Ristimäki A, Honkanen N, Jänkälä H, Sipponen P, Härkönen M. Expression of cyclooxygenase-2 in human gastric carcinoma. *Cancer Res.* 1997;57:1276–80.
29. Soydan AS, Gaffen JD, Weech PK, Tremblay NM, Kargman S, O'Neill G et al. Cytosolic phospholipase A$_2$, cyclo-oxygenases and arachidonate in human stomach tumours. *Eur J Cancer.* 1997;33:1508–12.
30. Mizuno H, Sakamoto C, Matsuda K, Wada K, Uchida T, Noguchi H et al. Induction of cyclooxygenase 2 in gastric mucosal lesions and its inhibition by the specific antagonist delays healing in mice. *Gastroenterology.* 1997;112:387–97.
31. Reuter BK, Asfaha S, Buret A, Sharkey KA, Wallace JL. Exacerbation of inflammation-associated colonic injury in rat through inhibition of cyclooxygenase-2. *J Clin Invest.* 1996;98:2076–85.

32. Sheng GG, Shao J, Sheng H, Hooton EB, Isakson PC, Morrow JD et al. A selective cyclooxygenase 2 inhibitor suppresses the growth of H-*ras*-transformed rat intestinal epithelial cells. *Gastroenterology.* 1997;113:1883–91.

33. Narko K, Ristimäki A, MacPhee M, Smith E, Haudenschild CC, Hla T. Tumorigenic transformation of immortalized ECV endothelial cells by cyclooxygenase-1 overexpression. *J Biol Chem.* 1997;272:21455–60.

34. Xie W, Chipman JG, Robertson DL, Erikson RL, Simmons DL. Expression of a mitogen-responsive gene encoding prostaglandin synthase is regulated by mRNA splicing. *Proc Natl Acad Sci USA.* 1991;88:2692–6.

35. Subbaramaiah K, Telang N, Ramonetti JT, Araki R, DeVito B, Weksler BB et al. Transcription of cyclooxygenase-2 is enhanced in transformed mammary epithelial cells. *Cancer Res.* 1996;56:4424–9.

36. Ristimäki A, Garfinkel S, Wessendorf J, Maciag T, Hla T. Induction of cyclooxygenase-2 by interleukin-1α. Evidence for post-transcriptional regulation. *J Biol Chem.* 1994;269:11769–75.

37. Ristimäki A, Narko K, Hla T. Down-regulation of cytokine-induced cyclooxygenase-2 transcript isoforms by dexamethasone: evidence for post-transcriptional regulation. *Biochem J.* 1996;318:325–31.

38. Sheng H, Shao J, Kirkland SC, Isakson P, Coffey RJ, Morrow J et al. Inhibition of human colon cancer cell growth by selective inhibition of cyclooxygenase-2. *J Clin Invest.* 1997;99:2254–9.

39. Tsuji S, Kawano S, Sawaoka H, Takei Y, Kobayashi I, Nagano K et al. Evidence for involvement of cyclooxygenase-2 in proliferation of two gastrointestinal cancer cell lines. *Prostaglandins Leukot Essent Fatty Acids.* 1996;55:179–83.

40. Tsujii M, DuBois RN. Alterations in cellular adhesion and apoptosis in epithelial cells overexpressing prostaglandin endoperoxide synthase 2. *Cell.* 1995;83:493–501.

41. Sheng H, Shao J, Morrow JD, Beauchamp RD, DuBois RN. Modulation of apoptosis and Bcl-2 expression by prostaglandin E_2 in human colon cancer cells. *Cancer Res.* 1998;58:362–6.

42. Müller-Deccer K, Scholz K, Marks F, Furstenberger G. Differential expression of prostaglandin H synthase isozymes during multistage carcinogenesis in mouse epidermis. *Mol Carcinog.* 1995;12:31–41.

43. Tsujii M, Kawano S, DuBois RN. Cyclooxygenase-2 expression in human colon cancer cells increases metastatic potential. *Proc Natl Acad Sci USA.* 1997;94:3336–40.

44. Hla T, Ristimäki A, Narko K, Ben-Av P, Lee M-J, Evans M et al. Role of the early response gene cyclooxygenase (COX)-2 in angiogenesis. In: Maragoudakis ME, editor. *Molecular, Cellular, and Clinical Aspects of Angiogenesis.* New York: Plenum Press; 1996:191–8.

45. Harada S-I, Nagy JA, Sullivan KA, Thomas KA, Endo N, Rodan GA et al. Induction of vascular endothelial growth factor expression by prostaglandin E_2 and E_1 in osteoblasts. *J Clin Invest.* 1994;93:2490–6.

46. Ben-Av P, Crofford LJ, Wilder RL, Hla T. Induction of endothelial growth factor expression in synovial fibroblasts by prostaglandin E and interleukin-1: a potential mechanism for inflammatory angiogenesis. *FEBS Lett.* 1995;372:83–7.

47. Majima M, Isono M, Ikeda Y, Hayashi I, Hatanaka K, Harada Y et al. Significant roles of inducible cyclooxygenase (COX)-2 in angiogenesis in rat sponge implants. *Jpn J Pharmacol.* 1997;75:105–14.

13

Suppression of intestinal polyposis by inhibition of cyclooxygenase-2 in a mouse model for familial adenomatous polyposis

M. M. TAKETO

Familial adenomatous polyposis (FAP) is a dominant disease that causes thousands of benign colonic polyps in the patient. If these polyps are left untreated, some of them eventually become malignant cancers. Currently, the major treatment for the disease is a prophylactic colectomy operation. However, such surgical procedures can seriously affect the quality of life, especially in young patients. Accordingly, it would be a tremendous benefit for the patient if the surgery could be postponed by drug treatment, even if only for 10 years. Through molecular genetic studies of FAP kindreds, the adenomatous polyposis coli (APC) gene on human chromosome 5q21 has been isolated and characterized[1-4]. Mutations in APC appear to be responsible not only for FAP but also for many sporadic cancers of the colorectal axis, as well as some stomach and oesophageal cancers[5-7]. APC consists of 15 coding exons and several 5′ noncoding exons, various combinations of which generate many isoforms by alternative splicing[3,8,9]. The gene encodes a huge protein of about 2840 aa[1,4]. The protein contains regions that may form an α-helical coiled-coil structure, and a subdomain of the first 55 aa form a stable, parallel helical dimer[10]. Antibody studies showed that the wild-type, but not mutant, APC protein is associated with the microtubule cytoskeleton[11,12]. The predicted structure of APC, its localization, and its interaction with β-catenin[13,14] suggested its involvement in cell adhesion. In fact, recent studies demonstrated that APC is localized to plasma membrane sites involved in active cell migration[15], and also in the nucleus[16]. At the same time, β-catenin interacts with hTcf-4 and Lef transcription factors. hTcf-4 transactivates transcription only when associated with β-catenin[17,18], suggesting the involvement of APC in cell signalling and transcriptional regulation.

MOUSE MODEL FOR FAP

To investigate the molecular mechanism of polyp formation followed by carcinogenesis in the digestive tract, an animal model of human FAP was developed. Taking advantage of gene targeting technology, we constructed an *Apc* gene knockout mouse strain that carried a truncation mutation at codon 716 ($Apc^{\Delta716}$)[19]. Although the homozygous mutant embryos died in utero before day eight of gestation, the heterozygotes were viable and developed multiple polyps throughout the intestinal tract, mostly in the small intestine. The earliest polyps arose multifocally during the third week after birth, and new polyps continued to appear thereafter. Interestingly, every nascent polyp in the small intestine consisted of a microadenoma covered with a layer of normal villous epithelium. These microadenomas originated from single crypts by formation of abnormal outpockets into the inner (lacteal) side of the neighbouring villi. We carefully dissected such microadenomas from nascent polyps by peeling off the normal epithelium and determined their genotype by PCR: all microadenomas had already lost the wild-type allele, whereas the mutant allele remained unchanged. These results indicate that loss of heterozygosity (LOH) followed by formation of intravillous microadenomas is responsible for the polyp adenoma initiation in the $Apc^{\Delta716}$ intestinal mucosa.

POLYP GROWTH MECHANISM IN $Apc^{\Delta716}$

We then analysed the processes of polyp development both at morphological and molecular levels[20]. The initiation process of a microadenoma can be explained by the cell migration defect in the proliferative zone cells that are devoid of the wild-type APC protein. Thus, a small intestinal microadenoma became initiated as an outpocketing pouch in a single crypt and developed into the inner (lacteal) side of an adjoining villus, forming a double-layer nascent polyp. The microadenoma then enlarged and became folded inside the villus. When it filled the intravillous space, it expanded downwards and extended into adjoining villi, rather than rupturing into the intestinal lumen. During the course of this development, the basement membrane remained intact, and the labelling index of the microadenoma cells was similar to that of the normal crypt epithelium. As in the crypt cell, neither transforming growth factor β1 nor its receptor type II was expressed in the adenoma cell. No hot spot mutations in the K-*ras* gene were found in the microadenoma tissue during these early stages of polyp development. Essentially the same results were obtained for the colonic polyps[20]. These results suggest that early adenomas in the $Apc^{\Delta716}$ polyps are very similar to the normal proliferating cells of the crypt except for the lack of directed migration along the crypt–villus axis. As in human FAP, the adenomas that develop in

$Apc^{\Delta 716}$ knockout mice are mostly benign adenomas, and submucosal invasions of the tumours are very rarely seen by the time these mice become moribund due to anaemia and dehydration at the age of 16–20 weeks[19].

The $Apc^{\Delta 716}$ mice provided a useful model for investigation of various carcinogens, and for evaluation of anticancer and chemopreventive agents. Earlier, we demonstrated that heterocyclic amines that are generated in over-cooked meat stimulate the growth of the intestinal polyps, whereas docosahexaenoic acid reduces the number of polyps significantly when fed to $Apc^{\Delta 716}$ mice[21,22]. Recently, we studied extensively the effect of cyclooxygenase 2 (COX-2) inhibition in $Apc^{\Delta 716}$ mice, as described below.

NSAIDS AND COLORECTAL TUMOURS

Cyclooxygenase (COX) plays a key role in arachidonate metabolism, as it catalyses biosynthesis of prostaglandin H_2, the precursor for prostanoids such as prostaglandins, prostacyclin and thromboxane[23,24]. In addition to COX-1, which was the first COX to be described and which is constitutively expressed in many tissues[25], a second isoenzyme, COX-2, was identified in 1991[26-29]. COX-2 is induced by various stimuli such as mitogens and cytokines, and is involved in many inflammatory reactions. Because non-steroidal anti-inflammatory drugs (NSAIDs) such as aspirin, indomethacin and sulindac inhibit both COX-1 and COX-2, they also cause unwanted side effects exemplified by gastrointestinal bleeding and ulceration[23,30].

Accumulating evidence indicates that NSAIDs reduce the incidence of colorectal cancers in humans and experimental animals, and reduce the polyp number and size in FAP patients[31]. For example, subcutaneous inoculation of Sprague–Dawley rats with methylazoxymethanol (MAM) at 10 weekly intervals caused about 20 tumours in the intestine after 20 weeks of treatment[32]. When indomethacin was given to the rats in drinking water two or 11 weeks after a single dose of MAM, the tumour incidence, multiplicity and size were reduced significantly[33]. These and other animal experiments demonstrated significant reduction in the incidence and multiplicity of colon tumours, and this effect was observed even after many weeks of carcinogen treatment.

In numerous retrospective and prospective epidemiological studies, on the other hand, the relative risk of developing colon cancer was significantly lower in patients (or sample population) taking aspirin or other NSAIDs. In elaborate studies in which the dosage and/or duration of NSAIDs intake were investigated, dose-dependent and/or duration-dependent reductions in the relative risk were often found[34,35].

In addition, both uncontrolled and randomized, controlled trials of sulindac in FAP patients demonstrated statistically significant reductions in both the number and size of polyps. However, there was a tendency for recurring polyps, in both the number and size, after sulindac was discontinued. Accordingly, the sulindac treatment in preoperative FAP patients was not sufficient to replace a colectomy operation, whereas it may be useful as an adjunct in postoperative cases[36,37]. One of the problems often faced in sulindac treatment of FAP patients appears to be severe side effects common to NSAIDs, such as gastrointestinal bleeding and ulceration. Although some patients tolerate sulindac without such problems, it can even be fatal in others. Because of this, there is a great need for new therapeutic agents such as COX-2 selective inhibitors.

COX-2 INDUCTION IN COLORECTAL CANCER

After the discovery of COX-2, studies of NSAIDs in cancers were focused on their relationship with COX-2 induction. In 1994, Eberhart et al.[38] reported that in 14 human colorectal carcinoma samples, 12 (86%) had marked increases in COX-2 mRNA, whereas 6 of 14 adenomas (43%) showed significant levels of COX-2 mRNA induction. In contrast, COX-1 mRNA levels were essentially the same in both adenomas and adenocarcinomas[38]. By immunoblot determination, Kargman et al.[39] showed that 19 of 25 (76%) human colon cancer tissues had significant levels of COX-2 induction, whereas no such induction was observed with matched normal colonic tissues. However, four premalignant polyps did not show such COX-2 induction[40]. Using an immunohistochemical method, Sano et al.[40] demonstrated that 15 human colorectal cancer tissues had marked COX-2 expression in cancer cells, inflammatory cells, vascular endothelium, and fibroblasts compared with the nonlesional, normal colon tissues. In contrast, expression of COX-1 protein was weak in both normal and cancer specimens[40]. Likewise, Kutchera et al.[41] found by in situ hybridization that the neoplastic colonocytes had increased expression of COX-2. Additionally, five colon cancer cell lines were shown to express high levels of COX-2 mRNA. By transfection experiments with the 5' regulatory sequence of the COX-2 gene ligated to a luciferase reporter, they found that colon cancer cell line HCT-116 constitutively expressed COX-2 whereas normal control cell lines transcribed the reporter only in response to an exogenous agonist[41].

COX-2 INDUCTION IN *Apc*$^{\Delta716}$ POLYPS

Accordingly, we determined expression of COX-2 in polyps which developed in *Apc*$^{\Delta716}$ mice. Immunoblot analyses of polyp proteins were performed using specific antibodies against COX-1 and COX-2. The normal intestinal epithelium, as well as polyps of various sizes expressed COX-1 protein at similar levels, in both the colon and small intestine. In contrast, the normal epithelium of neither the small intestine nor the colon contained any detectable COX-2 protein. However, polyps as small as 2 mm in diameter, either from the colon or small intestine, contained significant levels of COX-2 protein. The results indicate that COX-2 is induced in the polyp tissues at a very early stage of development, long before their malignant progression[42]. These results suggest that COX-2 may play an important role in polyp development, although they do not prove the thesis.

COX-2 GENE KNOCKOUT IN $Apc^{\Delta716}$ MICE

To investigate the effect of COX-2 on $Apc^{\Delta716}$ polyp formation, we introduced a knockout mutation of the COX-2 gene $(Ptgs2)$[43] into the $Apc^{\Delta716}$ knockout mice by successive crosses, and constructed compound mutant mice that carried $Apc^{\Delta716}$ (+/−) $Ptgs2$ (+/−) and $Apc^{\Delta716}$ (+/−) $Ptgs2$ (−/−) mutations, respectively. The $Apc^{\Delta716}$ (+/−) $Ptgs2$ (+/+) littermates were used as positive controls. When the intestinal polyps were scored at the same age, the polyp numbers in the $Apc^{\Delta716}$ (+/−) $Ptgs2$ (+/−) and $Apc^{\Delta716}$ (+/−) $Ptgs2$ (−/−) mice were reduced to 34% and 14% of the controls, respectively (Figure 1a). Moreover, the sizes of the polyps in these mice were significantly smaller than in the controls (Figure 1b). These results are the first direct genetic evidence that COX-2 plays a key role in polyp formation, and suggest that COX-2 inactivation suppresses polyp growth, rather than the initiation process[40]. This is in clear contrast with the effects of diets on $Apc^{\Delta716}$ polyps. We recently fed $Apc^{\Delta716}$ mice either low-fat and high-fibre diet (LRD for low-risk diet) or high-fat and low-fibre diet (HRD for high-risk diet) for seven weeks. Although the mice fed HRD developed polyps in significantly higher numbers than those fed LRD, in both the small intestine and colon, there was essentially no difference in the polyp size distribution between the two groups. It is likely that HRD increases the frequency of the initial event, i.e. LOH of the Apc gene[44].

Figure 1 Effects of Ptgs2 mutations on intestinal polyps in $Apc^{\Delta716}$ (+/−) Ptgs2 (+/−) and $Apc^{\Delta716}$ (+/−) Ptgs2 (/−) mice, compared with the $Apc^{\Delta716}$ (1/−) Ptgs2 (+/+) controls. (a) The mean numbers of polyps per mouse are shown with S.D. (b) Size distribution of the intestinal polyps. Polyp sizes were classified according to their diameters in mm. Reproduced with permission from reference 42.

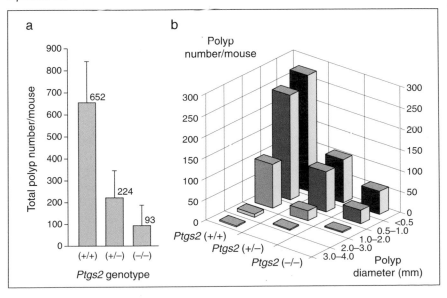

COX-2-SELECTIVE INHIBITOR ON *Apc*$^{\Delta716}$ MICE

In order to determine whether we could mimic the polyp-reducing effects of the COX-2 gene knockout mutation by administration of pharmaceutical agents to the *Apc*$^{\Delta716}$ mice, we tested the effects of a novel COX-2 selective inhibitor, MF tricyclic, and a nonselective COX inhibitor, sulindac. MF tricyclic is a research compound (Figure 2a) that is about 100-fold more selective against COX-2 than sulindac (Figure 2b). When fed at 14 and 3.5 mg/kg/day for eight weeks, MF tricyclic reduced the polyp numbers by 62% and 50% of the controls, respectively, compared with only 26% reduction by sulindac at 14 mg/kg/day (Figure 2c)[42]. These results indicate that the COX-2 selective inhibitor, MF tricyclic, is much more effective in reducing polyp number than the nonselective COX inhibitor sulindac, in addition to the very few gastrointestinal side effects of the COX-2 selective inhibitor.

COX-2 EXPRESSION IN *Apc*$^{\Delta716}$ TUMOUR STROMA

Interestingly, suppression of the COX-2 activity, either by introduction of the *Ptgs2* knockout mutation or by the COX-2 selective inhibitor, MF tricyclic, caused a profound effect on the polyp morphology as well. Well-developed polyps in the *Apc*$^{\Delta716}$ (+/−) *Ptgs2* (−/−) mouse intestine appeared recessed from the surface of the surrounding villi. This was essentially due to less stromal (i.e. interstitial) cells compared with the *Apc*$^{\Delta716}$ (+/−) *Ptgs2* (+/+) polyps[43]. To determine the site of COX-2 expression in the polyps, we constructed another strain of *Ptgs2* knockout mice in which one of the *Ptgs2* alleles was interrupted by a bacterial β-galactosidase gene (*lacZ*), placing *lacZ* under the control of the *Ptgs2* promoter. When this mutation was introduced into the *Apc*$^{\Delta716}$ mice [*Apc*$^{\Delta716}$ (+/−) *Ptgs2*^{lacZ} (+/−)], *lacZ* expression was found essentially in the stromal cells[42]. These results strongly suggest that the polyp adenoma grows through interactions between the epithelial and the stromal components, reminiscent of many processes of organogenesis in ontogeny[45]. To determine further the cell types that express COX-2 in the polyp tumour stroma, we performed an immuno-electron microscopic analysis. Bacterial β-galactosidase, the product of *LacZ* driven by the COX-2 promoter-enhancer was detected essentially in three types of cells: fibroblasts (Figure 3a), vascular endothelial cells (Figure 3b) and macrophages. Accordingly, it is conceivable that COX-2 expressed in the polyp stromal cells plays several different roles. For example, fibroblasts may secrete growth factors that stimulate tumour epithelium, whereas endothelial cells may be stimulated for angiogenesis by COX-2.

IS COX-2 A NEW PARADIGM IN CANCER?

These results have several implications and present important questions for future research, as pointed out by Prescott and White[46]. In the laboratory: (1) How does COX-2 expression become dysregulated after loss of APC function? (2) Is it

Figure 2 Effect of a novel COX-2 inhibitor MF tricyclic, and sulindac on Apc$^{\Delta 716}$ (+/–) mouse intestinal polyps. (a) Structure of MF tricyclic. (b) Structure of sulindac. (c) Number of polyps per mouse scored in Apc$^{\Delta 716}$ (+/–) mice fed with the control diet, or diet with MF tricyclic or sulindac. Circles indicate polyp numbers for individual females whereas squares indicate males. The number and vertical bar to the right of each sample group indicate the mean polyp number and S.D., respectively. The drug doses have been calculated from the concentrations of the drugs in the diet and the actual diet intakes. Reproduced with permission from reference 42.

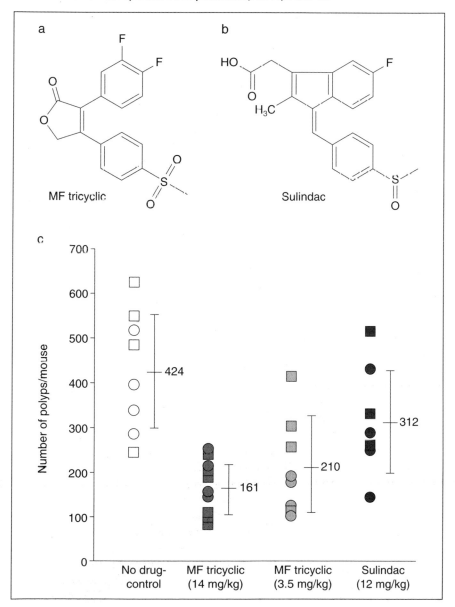

Figure 3 Immuno-electron microscopical analysis of LacZ protein expressed from the Ptgs2 promoter in the stromal cells of an intestinal polyp developed in the Apc$^{\Delta716}$ (+/–) Ptgs2^{LacZ} (+/–) mouse. (a) A fibroblast stained. Asterisks (*) show the nucleus and the cytoplasm. (b) Vascular endothelial cells are stained (asterisks;*). Scale bars: 1 μm.

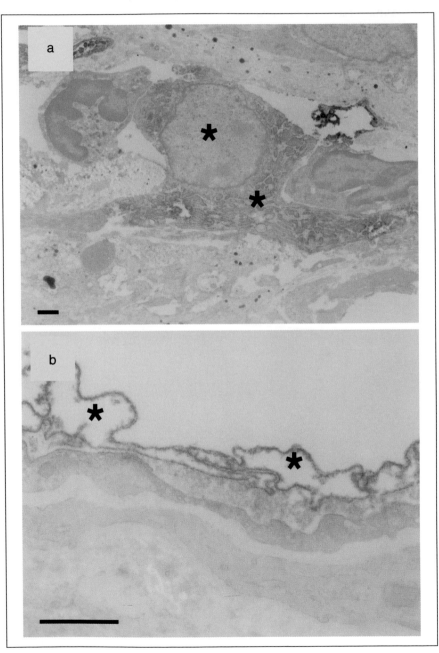

transcriptional, and if so, through which factors? (3) Is COX-2 expression alone sufficient to cause colon neoplasia? (4) What are the important products and what is the signalling pathway? (5) Which cellular responses lead to tumours (e.g. loss of apoptosis, others)? In the clinic: (1) Will specific inhibitors of COX-2 be more effective than non-selective NSAIDs? (2) Will inhibition of COX-2 be as effective in sporadic polyps and hereditary nonpolyposis colon cancer (HNPCC) as in FAP patients? (3) What accounts for the residual cases of neoplasia – is it a rare event that occurs only in some early polyps, or will all of them eventually escape the inhibitory effect? (4) How should chemoprevention with COX inhibitors be integrated into current surveillance and intervention protocols[46]?

With new COX-2 selective inhibitors of clinical grade, many new animal experiments and clinical trials will be performed in the coming years to determine their efficacy in chemotherapy for polyposis and various cancers, as well as cancer chemoprevention. Before rushing into clinical trials of all kinds of cancers, however, it would be important to determine whether COX-2 is induced and playing a key role in each type of cancer and/or pre-cancerous condition. Once this correlation is established, we can reasonably expect that treatments with COX-2 selective inhibitors will bring us promising chemotherapeutic effects.

Acknowledgements

I am grateful to the following colleagues who contributed to the work referred to in this review: Minoru Matsui, Masanobu Oshima, Hiroko Oshima, Kyoko Kitagawa, Masahiko Kobayashi, Susumu Nishimura, Masahiro Tsutsumi, Mami Takahashi, Keiji Wakabayashi, Minako Nagao, Takashi Sugimura, Kazunaga Yazawa and Kyoji Hioki (Japan); Joseph E Dinchuk, James M Trzaskos, Narayan Shivapurkar and Oliver Alabaster (USA); and Stacia L Kargman, Bruno Hancock, Elizabeth Kwong and Jilly F Evans (Canada). Also I thank the Cell Press for permission to reproduce the contents of the original paper in this article.

REFERENCES

1. Kinzler KW, Nilbert MC, Su L-K, Vogelstein B, Bryan TM, Levy DB et al. Identification of FAP locus genes from chromosome 5q21. *Science*. 1991;253:661–5.
2. Nishisho I, Nakamura Y, Miyoshi Y, Miki Y, Ando H, Horii A et al. Mutations of chromosome 5q21 genes in FAP and colorectal cancer patients. *Science*. 1991;253:665–9.
3. Groden J, Thliveris A, Samowitz W, Carlson M, Gelbert L, Albertsen H et al. Identification and characterization of the familial adenomatous polyposis coli gene. *Cell*. 1991;66:589–600.
4. Joslyn G, Carlson M, Thliveris A, Albertsen H, Gelbert L, Samowitz W et al. Identification of deletion mutations and three new genes at the familial polyposis locus. *Cell*. 1991;66:601–13.
5. Boynton RF, Blout PL, Yin J, Brown VL, Huang Y, Tong Y et al. Loss of heterozygosity involving the APC and MCC genetic loci occurs in the majority of human esophageal cancers. *Proc Natl Acad Sci USA*. 1992;89:3385–8.
6. Powell SM, Zilz N, Beazer-Barclay Y, Bryan TM, Hamilton SR, Thibodeau SN et al. APC mutations occur early during colorectal tumorigenesis. *Nature*. 1992;359:235–7.

7. Horii A, Nakatsuru S, Miyoshi Y, Ichii S, Ngase H, Kato K et al. The APC gene, responsible for familial adenomatous polyposis, is mutated in human gastric cancer. *Cancer Res.* 1992;52:3231–3.

8. Oshima M, Sugiyama H, Kitagawa K, Taketo M. APC gene messenger RNA: novel isoforms that lack exon 7. *Cancer Res.* 1993;53:5589–91.

9. Thliveris A, Samowitz W, Matunami N, Groden J, White R. Demonstration of promoter activity and alternative splicing in the region 5' to exon 1 of the APC gene. *Cancer Res.* 1994;54:2991–5.

10. Joslyn G, Richardson DS, White R, Alber T. Dimer formation by and N-terminal coiled coil in the APC protein. *Proc Natl Acad Sci USA.* 1993;90:11109–13.

11. Smith KJ, Levy DB, Maupin P, Pollard TD, Vogelstein B, Kinzler KW. Wild-type but not mutant APC associates with the microtubule cytoskeleton. *Cancer Res.* 1994;54:3672–5.

12. Munemitsu S, Souza B, Müller O, Albert I, Rubinfeld B, Polakis P. The APC gene product associates with microtubules in vivo and promotes their assembly in vitro. *Cancer Res.* 1994;54:3676–81.

13. Rubinfeld B, Souza B, Albert B, Müller O, Chamberlain SH, Masiarz FR et al. Association of the APC gene product with β-catenin. *Science.* 1993;262:1731–4.

14. Su L-K, Vogelstein B, Kinzler KW. Association of the APC tumor suppressor protein with catenins. *Science.* 1993;262:1734–7.

15. Nathke IS, Adams CL, Polakis P, Sellin JH, Nelson WJ. The adenomatous polyposis coli tumor suppressor protein localizes to plasma membrane sites involved in active cell migration. *J Cell Biol.* 1996;134:165–78.

16. Neufeld KL, White RL. Nuclear and cytoplasmic localization of the adenomatous polyposis coli protein. *Proc Natl Acad Sci USA.* 1997;94:3034–9.

17. Korinek V, Barker N, Morin PJ, van Wichen D, de Weger R, Kinzler KW et al. Constitutive transcriptional activation by a β-catenin-Tcf complex in APC–/– colon carcinoma. *Science.* 1997;275:1784–7.

18. Morin PJ, Sparks AB, Korinek V, Barker N, Clevers H, Vogelstein B, Kinzler KW. Activation of β-catenin-Tcf signaling in colon cancer by mutations in β-catenin or APC. *Science.* 1997;275:1787–90.

19. Oshima M, Oshima H, Kitagawa K, Kobayashi M, Itakura C, Taketo M. Loss of *Apc* heterozygosity and abnormal tissue building in nascent intestinal polyps in mice carrying a truncation *Apc* gene. *Proc Natl Acad Sci USA.* 1995;92:4482–6.

20. Oshima H, Oshima M, Kobayashi M, Tsutsumi M, Taketo MM. Morphological and molecular polyp formation in *Apc*$^{\Delta716}$ knockout mice. *Cancer Res.* 1997;57:1644–9.

21. Oshima M, Oshima H, Tsutsumi M, Nishimura S, Sugimura T, Nagao M et al. Effects of 2-amino-1-methyl-6-phenylimidazo[4,5-*b*]pyridine on intestinal polyp development in *Apc*$^{\Delta716}$ knockout mice. *Mol Carcinog.* 1996;15:11–17.

22. Oshima M, Takahashi M, Oshima H, Tsutsumi M, Yazawa K, Sugimura T et al. Effects of docosahexaenoic acid (DHA) on intestinal polyp development in *Apc*$^{\Delta716}$ knockout mice. *Carcinogenesis.* 1995;16:2605–7.

23. Vane JR. Inhibition of prostaglandin synthesis as a mechanism of action for aspirin-like drugs. *Nature New Biol.* 1971;231:232–5.

24. Vane J. Towards a better aspirin. *Nature.* 1994;367:215–6.

25. O'Neill GP, Ford-Hutchinson AW. Expression of mRNA for cyclooxygenase-1 and cyclooxygenase-2 in human tissues. *FEBS Lett.* 1993;330:156–60.

26. Maier JAM, Hla T, Maciag H. Cyclooxygenase is an immediate-early gene induced by interleukin-1 in human endothelial cells. *J Biol Chem.* 1990;265:10805–8.

27. Lee SH, Soyoola E, Chanmugam P, Hart S, Sun W, Zhong H et al. Selective expression of mitogen-inducible cyclooxygenase in macrophages stimulated with lipopolysaccharide. *J Biol Chem.* 1992;267:25934–8.

28. O'Banion MK, Winn VD, Young DA. cDNA cloning and functional activity of a glucocorticoid-regulated inflammatory cyclooxygenase. *Proc Natl Acad Sci USA*. 1992;89:4888–92.

29. Xie W, Robertson DL, Simmons DL. Mitogen-inducible prostaglandin G/H synthase: a new target for nonsteroidal antiinflammatory drugs. *Drug Dev Res*. 1992;25:249–65.

30. Mitchell JA, Akarasereenont P, Thiemermann C, Flower RJ, Vane JR. Selectivity of non-steroidal antiinflammatory drugs as inhibitors of constitutive and inducible cyclooxygenase. *Proc Natl Acad Sci USA*. 1993;90:11693–7.

31. Marnett LJ. Aspirin and the potential role of prostaglandins in colon cancer. *Cancer Res*. 1992;52:5575–89.

32. Pollard M, Zederck MS. Induction of colon tumors in 1,2-dimethylhydrazine-resistant Lobund Wistar rats by methylazoxymethanol acetate. *J Natl Cancer Inst*. 1978;61:493–4.

33. Pollard M, Luckert PH. Prolonged antitumor effects of indomethacin on autochthonous intestinal tumors in rats. *J Natl Cancer Inst*. 1983;70:1103–5.

34. Peleg II, Maiboch HT, Brown SH, Wilcox CM. Aspirin and non-steroidal anti-inflammatory drug use and the risk of subsequent colorectal cancer. *Arch Int Med*. 1994;154:394–9.

35. Giovannucci E, Rimm EB, Stampfer MJ, Colditz GA, Ascherio A, Willett WC. Aspirin use and the risk for colorectal cancer and adenoma in male health professionals. *Ann Intern Med*. 1994;121:241–6.

36. Giardiello FM, Hamilton SR, Krush AJ, Piantadosi S, Hylind LM, Celano P et al. Treatment of colonic and rectal adenomas with sulindac in familial adenomatous polyposis. *N Engl J Med*. 1993;328:1313–6.

37. Nugent KP, Farmer KC, Spigelman AD, Williams CB, Phillips RK. Randomized control trial of the effect of sulindac on duodenal and rectal polyposis and cell proliferation in patients with familial adenomatous polyposis. *Br J Surg*. 1993;80:1618–9.

38. Eberhart CE, Coffey RJ, Radhika A, Giardiello FM, Ferrenbach S, DuBois RN. Up-regulation of cyclooxygenase 2 gene expression in human colorectal adenomas and adenocarcinomas. *Gastroenterology*. 1994;107:1183–8.

39. Kargman SL, O'Neill GP, Vickers PJ, Evans JF, Mancini JA, Jothy S. Expression of prostaglandin G/H synthase-1 and -2 protein in human colon cancer. *Cancer Res*. 1995;55:2556–9.

40. Sano H, Kawahito Y, Wilder RL, Hashiramoto A, Mukai S, Asai K et al. Expression of cyclooxygenase-1 and -2 in human colorectal cancer. *Cancer Res*. 1995;55:3785–9.

41. Kutchera W, Jones DA, Matsunami N, Groden J, McIntyre TM, Zimmerman GA et al. Prostaglandin H synthase 2 is expressed abnormally in human colon cancer: evidence for a transcriptional effect. *Proc Natl Acad Sci USA*. 1996;93:4816–20.

42. Oshima M, Dinchuk JE, Kargman SL, Oshima H, Hancock B, Kwong E et al. Suppression of intestinal polyposis in $Apc^{\Delta716}$ knockout mice by inhibition of cyclooxygenase-2 (COX-2). *Cell*. 1996;87:803–9.

43. Dinchuk JE, Car BD, Focht RJ, Johnston JJ, Jaffee BD, Covington MB et al. Renal abnormalities and an altered inflammatory response in mice lacking cyclooxygenase II. *Nature*. 1995;378:406–9.

44. Hioki K, Shivapurkar N, Oshima H, Alabaster O, Oshima M, Taketo MM. Suppression of intestinal polyp development by low-fat and high-fiber diet in $Apc^{\Delta716}$ knockout mice. *Carcinogenesis*. 1997;18:1863–5.

45. Hong WK, Sporn MB. Recent advances in chemoprevention of cancer. *Science*. 1997;278:1073–7.

46. Prescott SM, White RL. Self promotion? Intimate connections between the tumor suppressor APC and prostaglandin H synthase-2 (COX-2). *Cell*. 1996;87:801–3.

14

Meloxicam inhibits the growth of colorectal cancer cells

A. P. GOLDMAN, C. S. WILLIAMS, L. W. LAMPS, V. P. WILLIAMS, M. PAIRET, J. D. MORROW AND R. N. DUBOIS

Colorectal cancer is the second leading cause of death from cancer in Western civilizations, claiming about 55,000–60,000 lives each year in the United States. Americans have a 1 in 20 lifetime risk of developing this disease and approximately 1 in 10 has a family member who develops colorectal cancer. Understanding the environmental and molecular events involved in the multi-step progression from normal epithelium to malignant transformation will be helpful in designing diagnostic tests and successful therapeutic interventions. Epidemiological studies evaluating large cohorts of individuals demonstrate that regular aspirin use leads to a 40–50% reduction in mortality from colorectal cancer[1-6]. Recent studies indicate that cyclooxygenase-2 (COX-2) levels are increased in approximately 85% of colorectal cancers[7] and COX-2 is a key enzyme required for prostaglandin synthesis. One of the known effects of non-steroidal anti-inflammatory drugs (NSAIDs) is their ability to inhibit COX enzymes.

The chemoprotective effects of NSAIDs are counterbalanced by the risk of gastrointestinal toxicity, which can be manifest as gastric ulceration and/or gastrointestinal bleeding. Gastrointestinal toxicity is thought to be due to inhibition of COX-1 which is present in the gastric mucosa[8]. Recently, several drug companies have developed agents which are highly selective inhibitors of COX-2 in the hope that these can produce analgesic benefits without associated gastrointestinal side effects. Evaluation of selective COX-2 inhibitors for effects on colorectal cancer is currently an area of intense investigation and pre-clinical studies have clearly shown potent antitumour properties associated with selective COX-2 inhibitors[9-12].

There is some controversy concerning the mechanism by which NSAIDs inhibit colorectal tumour growth[13,14]. It was recently demonstrated in both an in vitro and in vivo colorectal cancer model that a highly selective COX-2 inhibitor, SC-58125, reduced cell growth and tumour size[9]. If inhibiting COX-2 is the mechanism whereby NSAIDs decrease tumour size, then using another COX-2 inhibitor should yield similar results. Therefore, the aim of the present study was to determine if another (structurally unrelated) COX-2 inhibitor (meloxicam) has antitumour properties.

HCA-7, MOSER-S AND HCT-116 COLONY GROWTH IN MATRIGEL

To assess whether meloxicam is effective at inhibiting cell growth in vitro, HCA-7, Moser-S and HCT-116 cells were grown in MatriGel in the presence or absence of meloxicam. HCA-7 (a generous gift from S. Kirkland), Moser-S (provided by R. D. Beauchamp) and HCT-116 (ATCC #CCL 247) human colorectal cancer cell lines were selected for evaluation due to their different levels of COX-2 expression.

Neither of the COX-2-positive cell lines has detectable COX-1 protein as assessed by Western blot analysis. HCT-116 cells do not express either COX-1 or COX-2 protein by Western blot analysis. All cell lines were maintained in McCoy's 5M Modified Medium (Gibco, Inc., Grand Island, NY, USA) until they were ~90% confluent. Once a cell density of 1×10^5 HCA-7 cells/well, 5×10^4 HCT-116 cells/well and 5×10^4 Moser-S cells/well was achieved, the cells were suspended in 1:2 diluted MatriGel (Collaborative Biomedical Products, Bedford, MA, USA) in three separate 24-well plates. Lower densities of Moser-S and HCT-116 cells were plated due to their faster growth relative to HCA-7 cells. Following MatriGel solidification, 1.0 ml of McCoy's medium with 1, 5, 10, 25, 30, 50 or 100 μM meloxicam (Boehringer Ingelheim, Inc., Germany) was added to the wells of all cell types. Experimental controls were treated with dimethylsulphoxide (DMSO) alone. The medium, containing meloxicam at the indicated concentrations, was replaced daily. On day 14, each well was photographed three times with a camera attached to the microscope at a magnification of 4×. Relative colony size was determined by measuring 10 random colonies from each slide (30 measurements/well). Means for each dose were calculated and compared to controls[15].

A dose-dependent decrease in colony size was observed in HCA-7 and Moser-S cells following daily administration of meloxicam (1–100 μM). Meloxicam treatment significantly reduced the size of HCA-7 colonies, with a greater effect at higher concentrations ($P<0.01$). On day 14, HCA-7 colonies treated with 1 μM meloxicam were 72% smaller than controls and those treated with 100 μM showed a 97% decrease in volume (Table 1). A significant effect, though less dramatic, was observed in the Moser-S cells (Table 1). Meloxicam did not have a significant effect on colony volume in HCT-116 cells, which do not express COX-2 protein. The mean colony number was reduced by 20% in

Table 1 Effect of meloxicam on HCA-7, Moser-S and HCT-116 colony formation

Cell line	Meloxicam (μM)	Relative colony volume (compared to controls)
HCA-7	0	1.00
	1	0.28
	5	0.28
	10	0.32
	25	0.24
	30	0.17
	50	0.11
	100	0.03
Moser-S	0	1.00
	5	0.71
	10	0.67
	25	0.43
HCT-116	0	1.00
	5	0.76
	10	0.76
	25	0.76

HCA-7, Moser-S and HCT-116 cells were grown in triplicate wells of MatriGel for 14 days in either the absence (with DMSO) or presence of meloxicam at the indicated concentrations. Prior to the analysis of PGE_2 levels in the medium, medium was changed to serum-free containing the indicated meloxicam concentrations and supplemented with 10 μM arachidonic acid for 1 hour. On day 14, the cultures were photographed in three separate fields and the sizes of 10 random colonies were measured. The data are shown as the mean colony size of the treated samples relative to the appropriate control.

HCA-7 cells and by 22% in Moser-S cells treated with 25 μM meloxicam (P=0.003 and 0.032 respectively). In contrast, no dose-dependent reduction in colony number was observed in HCT-116 cells (Table 1).

PROSTAGLANDIN SYNTHESIS IN CULTURED CELLS

The effectiveness of meloxicam in inhibiting the synthesis of prostaglandin E_2 (PGE_2) was determined in both control and treated cells by measuring PGE_2 levels in the medium. PGE_2 is the predominant prostaglandin product of HCA-7 cells and it has been previously reported that COX-2 inhibitors, such as SC-58125 and NS-398, are effective in inhibiting PGE_2 production in these cells[9,16]. HCA-7, Moser-S and HCT-116 cells were treated with 1, 5, 10 or 25 μM meloxicam for 23 hours, at which time the medium was replaced with serum-free medium containing meloxicam at the concentrations indicated plus 10 μM arachidonic acid for 1 hour. PGE_2 in the medium taken from the cells was measured (in triplicate) at each meloxicam dose. PGE_2 was measured using stable isotope dilution techniques with gas chromatography negative ion chemical ionization mass spectrometry as previously described[7].

Compared with the controls, PGE_2 levels in the meloxicam-treated HCA-7 cells were decreased by 92% with 1 μM meloxicam. A further reduction to 96% was noted with 5, 10 and 25 μM of meloxicam ($P<0.003$ for all doses) (Table 2). As in the HCA-7 cells, PGE_2 levels in medium taken from Moser-S cells were decreased by 72% with 1 μM meloxicam and by 86% with 25 μM meloxicam ($P<0.0193$ for all doses). It is important to note that PGE_2 levels at baseline were approximately 90% lower in the Moser-S cells than in the HCA-7 cells. This is likely to be due to a relatively low level of COX-2 enzyme detected in the Moser-S cells. Because there is no detectable COX-1 or COX-2 protein found in HCT-116 cells, we did not detect measurable levels of PGE_2 (data not shown).

COX-1 AND COX-2 EXPRESSION IN HCA-7 CELLS

In an attempt to determine if meloxicam treatment altered the expression of COX-1 or COX-2, Western blot analysis was performed on HCA-7 protein extracts. Since the greatest effect of meloxicam was observed in the HCA-7 cells, we evaluated COX-1 and COX-2 protein levels in these cells. HCA-7 cells were grown in 100 mm plates until 90% confluent, then treated with 50 μM meloxicam for 2, 4, 8, 12, 24 and 48 hours before harvesting and isolation of the protein extracts for Western blot analysis.

Immunoblot analyses of HCA-7 cell lysates were performed as previously described[7]. Briefly, the cultured HCA-7 cells were prepared in RIPA buffer containing 150 mM sodium chloride, 1% Nonidet P-40, 0.5% sodium deoxycholate and 0.1% sodium dodecyl sulphate (SDS) in water for 30 minutes. Protein samples (50 μg) were denatured in sample buffer and fractionated by 7.5% SDS-polyacrylamide gel electrophoresis (SDS-PAGE), after which the proteins were

Table 2 Effect of meloxicam on PGE_2 levels in HCA-7 and Moser-S cells

Cell line	Meloxicam (μM)	PGE_2 (ng/ml)
HCA-7	0	8.987
	1	0.681
	5	0.334
	10	0.337
	25	0.325
Moser-S	0	0.883
	1	0.250
	5	0.133
	10	0.107
	25	0.123

HCA-7 and Moser-S cells were grown to 90% confluence in serum-containing medium in either the absence (with DMSO) or presence of meloxicam (1–25 μM). Prior to the analysis of PGE_2 levels, the medium was changed to serum-free containing the indicated meloxicam concentrations and supplemented with 10 μM arachidonic acid for 1 hour. All measurements were done in triplicate.

transferred to PVDF membranes. After processing, the membranes were probed with either antihuman COX-1 or antihuman COX-2 antibodies (Santa Cruz Biotechnology Inc., Santa Cruz, CA, USA). The immune complexes were detected using horseradish peroxidase (HRP)-conjugated secondary antibodies and enhanced chemiluminescence (ECL) (Amersham, Arlington Heights, IL, USA). MC-26 and HCA-7 (untreated) cells were used as a positive control for COX-1 and COX-2, respectively, and the COX-1 and COX-2 null cells, HCT-116, were used as a negative control for Western analysis. The blots were washed and incubated with the ECL chemiluminescence system and then autoradiography was performed with Hyperfilm ECL (Amersham).

COX-1 protein was undetectable in 50 μg of HCA-7 cell lysate at the exposure times indicated (Table 3). In contrast, HCA-7 cells expressed relatively high levels of COX-2 protein and treatment with meloxicam led to a significant decrease in COX-2 following 24 hours of treatment (Table 3). Therefore, in addition to inhibiting COX enzyme activity, meloxicam treatment reduces COX-2 expression in HCA-7 cells.

TUMOUR GROWTH IN NUDE MICE

After demonstrating that meloxicam treatment of HCA-7 cells inhibits PGE₂ production and colony growth, we evaluated the effect of meloxicam on growth of HCA-7 cells in vivo.

Twelve athymic mice (Harlan Sprague Dawley, Inc., Indianapolis, IN, USA) were housed (12 hour light: 12 hour darkness schedule) in autoclave-sterilized cages and were provided with sterile food and water. Five mice were designated

Table 3 Western analysis of COX-1 and COX-2 in HCA-7 cells treated with meloxicam for various lengths of time

Hours of meloxicam exposure (50 μM)	COX-2 level	COX-1 level
0	++++	−
2	++++	−
4	+++	−
8	+++++	−
12	+++	−
24	++	−
48	+	−

HCA-7 cells were treated with 50 μM meloxicam for 0 to 48 hours in order to evaluate COX-1 and COX-2 expression. Protein extracts (50 μg) were separated by SDS-PAGE, transferred to PVDF and immunoblotted using either COX-1 or COX-2 specific antibodies. The immune complexes were detected using HRP-conjugated secondary antibodies and ECL. Extracts derived from MC-26 and HCA-7 (untreated) cells were used as a positive control for COX-1 and COX-2, respectively, and protein extracts from the HCT-116 cells were used as a negative control. COX-1 and COX-2 co-migrate with the pre-stained 68 kDa molecular mass marker.

as controls and the remaining seven mice assigned to the treatment group. Just before HCA-7 cell inoculation, the treatment group was given 40 mg/kg of meloxicam by intraperitoneal (i.p.) injection. Following the meloxicam injection, 5×10^6 HCA-7 cells were suspended in 0.1 ml of phosphate-buffered saline and injected subcutaneously on the dorsal flank of each mouse. The treatment was continued at a dose of 20 mg/kg per injection twice daily. Length and width measurements of the tumours were made with a calliper according to published methods[17]. Tumour volume was calculated based on the equation $V=(L \times W^2)/2$, where V is volume, L is length and W is width. Following eight weeks of treatment, tumours were measured, harvested and fixed in 10% buffered formalin and routinely processed. Four-micron sections were prepared and stained with routine haematoxylin and eosin and examined by a pathologist (LWL) in a blinded fashion.

   Examination of the tumours from the mice confirmed that they were adeno-carcinomas with well-formed glands and focal mucin production. Treatment with meloxicam for three weeks significantly reduced tumour size ($P=0.047$). This trend continued throughout the remainder of the experiment, which was terminated following eight weeks of meloxicam administration (Table 4). At the conclusion of the experiment, the meloxicam-treated tumours were 52% smaller than control tumours. There was no significant difference between the histology of the treated tumours and those in the control group.

CONCLUSIONS

Epidemiological and animal studies suggest that NSAIDs have potent anti-tumour properties[1–6,18–22]. Most of the NSAIDs used in animal studies are non-selective inhibitors of COX, thus the relative role of COX-1 or COX-2 inhibition is unknown. Several strategies can be adopted for evaluating the relative contribution of either COX-1 or COX-2 to tumour biology: (1) genetic experiments mating animals prone to colorectal cancer with animals lacking the COX-1 or COX-2 gene, (2) manipulating the expression of either COX isoform in cell culture models and assessing the phenotypic changes of these cells, or (3) isoform-selective inhibition in a variety of tumour models. Each of these approaches has

Table 4 Treatment of HCA-7 xenografts with meloxicam

Group	Mean volume (mm³) (day 28)	Mean volume (mm³) (day 56)
Control	200.8	588.1
Meloxicam	97.6	281.7

HCA-7 cells (5×10^6) were injected under the dorsal skin of nude mice, and meloxicam (20 mg/kg) was injected i.p. twice daily beginning at the time of HCA-7 inoculation. The volumes of the xenografts were measured weekly, and after eight weeks of treatment the mice were sacrificed. Tumour volume was calculated using the equation $V=(L \times W^2)/2$. Five mice were allocated to in the control group and seven to the treated.

certain limitations, but studies employing a combination of these approaches have strongly implicated COX-2 in the promotion of intestinal tumourigenesis. Selective COX-2 inhibitors are being developed by a number of pharmaceutical companies. We previously reported that a selective COX-2 inhibitor (SC-58125) was effective in inhibiting the growth of COX-2-positive HCA-7 cells[9]. Treatment of COX-2-negative HCT-116 cells with SC-58125 did not affect tumour growth, suggesting that the effects of SC-58125 on HCA-7 cells were mediated through inhibition of COX-2.

If COX-2 is a relevant target of NSAIDs, then other (structurally unrelated) COX-2 inhibitors should also be effective in inhibiting tumour growth. To test this hypothesis we evaluated the effect of meloxicam, a COX-2 inhibitor, in both in vitro and in vivo tumour growth assays. We observed a significant reduction in colony size, indicating that meloxicam inhibits the growth of HCA-7 cells. Treatment of mice with mcloxicam resulted in a statistically significant reduction in size of HCA-7 tumour xenografts, and this supports the hypothesis that COX-2 is involved in regulation of tumour growth. The experiments described here, in agreement with our previous findings, indicate that selective inhibition of COX-2 can affect tumour growth and this supports the hypothesis that COX-2 may serve as an important molecular target for prevention and/or treatment of colorectal cancer in humans.

Acknowledgements

This work was supported by the Boehringer Ingelheim Pharmaceutical Company and the US Public Health Services Grants DK-47297 (RND), ES-00267 (RND), DK-48831 (JDM), GM-42056 (JDM), GM-15431 (JDM) and VA Merit Award (RND). We also thank Dr Rebecca Shattuck-Brandt for editorial assistance.

REFERENCES

1. Thun MJ, Namboodiri MM, Heath CWJ. Aspirin use and reduced risk of fatal colon cancer. *N Engl J Med*. 1991;325:1593–6.
2. Rosenberg L, Palmer J, Zauber A, Washauer M, Stolley P, Shapiro S. A hypothesis: Nonsteroidal anti-inflammatory drugs reduce the incidence of large-bowel cancer. *J Natl Cancer Inst*. 1991;83:355–8.
3. Suh O, Mettlin C, Petrelli NJ. Aspirin use, cancer, and polyps of the large bowel. *Cancer*. 1993;72:1171–7.
4. Logan RF, Little J, Hawkin PG, Hardcastle JD. Effect of aspirin and non-steroidal anti-inflammatory drugs on colorectal adenomas: case-control study of subjects participating in the Nottingham faecal occult blood screening programme. *Br Med J*. 1993;307:285–9.
5. Peleg II, Maibach HT, Brown SH, Wilcox CM. Aspirin and nonsteroidal anti-inflammatory drug use and the risk of subsequent colorectal cancer. *Arch Int Med*. 1994;154:394–9.
6. Muscat JE, Stellman SD, Wynder EL. Nonsteroidal antiinflammatory drugs and colorectal cancer. *Cancer*. 1994;74:1847–54.
7. DuBois RN, Radhika A, Reddy BS, Entingh AJ. Increased cyclooxygenase-2 levels in carcinogen-induced rat colonic tumors. *Gastroenterology*. 1996;110:1259–62.

8. Bedi A, Pasricha PJ, Akhtar AJ, Barber JP, Bedi GC, Giardiello FM et al. Inhibition of apoptosis during development of colorectal cancer. *Cancer Res*. 1995;55:1811–6.

9. Sheng H, Shao J, Kirkland SC, Isakson P, Coffey R, Morrow J et al. Inhibition of human colon cancer cell growth by selective inhibition of cyclooxygenase-2. *J Clin Invest*. 1997;99:2254–9.

10. Oshima M, Dinchuk JE, Kargman SL, Oshima H, Hancock B, Kwong E et al. Suppression of intestinal polyposis in APC$^{\Delta716}$ knockout mice by inhibition of prostaglandin endoperoxide synthase-2 (COX-2). *Cell*. 1996;87:803–9.

11. Reddy BS, Rao CV, Seibert K. Evaluation of cyclooxygenase-2 inhibitor for potential chemopreventive properties in colon carcinogenesis. *Cancer Res*. 1996;56:4566–9.

12. Kawamori T, Rao CV, Seibert K, Reddy BS. Chemopreventive activity of celecoxib a specific cyclooxygenase-2 inhibitor against colon carcinogenesis. *Cancer Res*. 1998;58:409–12.

13. Levy DB, Smith KJ, Beazer-Barclay Y, Hamilton SR, Vogelstein B, Kinzler KW. Inactivation of both APC alleles in human and mouse tumors. *Cancer Res*. 1994;54:5953–8.

14. Abramson SB, Weissman G. The mechanisms of action of antiinflammatory drugs. *Arthritis Rheum*. 1989;32:1–9.

15. DuBois RN, Shao J, Sheng H, Tsujii M, Beauchamp RD. G$_1$ delay in intestinal epithelial cells overexpressing prostaglandin endoperoxide synthase-2. *Cancer Res*. 1996;56:733–7.

16. Tsuji S, Kawano S, Sawaoka H, Takei Y, Kobayashi I, Nagano K et al. Evidences for involvement of cyclooxygenase-2 in proliferation of two gastrointestinal cancer cell lines. *Prostaglandins Leukot Essent Fatty Acids*. 1996;55:179–83.

17. Wang J, Sun L, Myeroff L, Wang X, Gentry LE, Yang J et al. Demonstration that mutation of the type II transforming growth factor beta receptor inactivates its tumor suppressor activity in replication error-positive colon carcinoma cells. *J Biol Chem*. 1995;270:22044–9.

18. Davis AE, Patterson F. Aspirin reduces the incidence of colonic carcinoma in the dimethylhydrazine rat animal model. *Aust N Z J Med*. 1994;24:301–3.

19. Wargovich MJ, Chen CD, Harris C, Yang E, Velasco M. Inhibition of aberrant crypt growth by non-steroidal anti-inflammatory agents and differentiation agents in the rat colon. *Int J Cancer*. 1995;60:515–9.

20. Beazer-Barclay Y, Levy DB, Moser AR, Dove WF, Hamilton SR, Vogelstein B et al. Sulindac suppresses tumorigenesis in the *Min* mouse. *Carcinogenesis*. 1996;17:1757–60.

21. Boolbol SK, Dannenberg AJ, Chadburn A, Martucci C, Guo XJ, Ramonetti JT et al. Cyclooxygenase-2 overexpression and tumor formation are blocked by sulindac in a murine model of familial adenomatous polyposis. *Cancer Res*. 1996;56:2556–60.

22. Jacoby RF, Marshall DJ, Newton MA, Novakovic K, Tutsch K, Cole CE et al. Chemoprevention of spontaneous intestinal adenomas in the Apc^{Min} mouse model by the nonsteroidal anti-inflammatory drug piroxicam. *Cancer Res*. 1996;56:710–4.

Adverse effects of non-steroidal anti-inflammatory drugs on the gastrointestinal tract and kidney: relationship to cyclooxygenase-2 selectivity

P. McGETTIGAN, D. HENRY AND J. PAGE

The serious adverse effects of the 'classical' non-steroidal anti-inflammatory drugs (NSAIDs) have been the subject of much research. The main 'predictable' adverse effects are gastrointestinal (GI) ulceration, with its complications of haemorrhage and perforation, the development of functional renal impairment and the precipitation of congestive heart failure in susceptible individuals[1-9]. Other adverse effects, including damage to the small intestine, large bowel haemorrhage and acute liver damage, are fairly well established, but of less epidemiological and clinical significance because of their lower incidence and severity. There is reasonable evidence that much of the significant predictable toxicity of these drugs is related to inhibition of cyclooxygenase (COX)-1. Drugs with high selectivity for COX-2 may be less prone to cause these adverse effects and this would be a substantial advance in the management of musculo-skeletal disease[10].

In this brief review, we look at the correlations between the epidemiological estimates of risk of serious GI and renal complications of therapy, and the evidence concerning COX-2 selectivity. Although, like others, we believe that COX-2 selective drugs may prove to be a significant advance in therapy, we caution that when interpreting epidemiological estimates of risk with the 'classical' non-selective NSAIDs, confounding by factors such as ingested dose and plasma half life makes it difficult to assess the independent effect of COX selectivity.

Table I Estimates of risk for upper GI complications

	Henry et al. 1993[1]		Garcia Rodriguez et al. 1994[2]	
Outcome	UGIB, perforation[a]		UGIB, perforation	
Type of study	Population-based, case-control study n = 644 cases, 1268 controls		Population-based, case-control study n = 1457 cases, 10,000 controls	
Estimated RR/OR: UGIB (95% CI)		UGIB/perforation OR (95% CI)	Current use No use Ibuprofen Naproxen Diclofenac Ketoprofen Indomethacin Multiple NSAIDs Piroxicam Azapropazone	RR UGIB 1.0 2.9 (1.7, 5.0) 3.1 (1.7, 5.9) 3.9 (2.3, 6.5) 5.4 (2.6, 11.3) 6.3 (3.3, 12.2) 8.9 (5.4, 14.7) 18.0 (8.2, 39.6) 23.4, (6.9, 79.5)
	Ibuprofen	0.7 (0.4, 2.4)		
	Diflunisal	1.0 (0.4, 2.4)		
	Diclofenac	1.7 (1.1, 2.5)		
	Sulindac	2.1 (1.1, 4.1)		
	Indomethacin	2.5 (1.5, 4.1)		
	Naproxen	2.8 (1.8, 4.3)		
	Ketoprofen	3.6 (2.0, 6.6)		
	Piroxicam	4.8 (2.6, 8.7)		
	Any NSAID, UGIB, alone: 2.8 (2.2, 3.5) Any NSAID, perforation: 6.1 (2.1, 17.9)			
Dose-response relation-ship	Doses[b] in previous week <2 ≥14	OR (95% CI) 2.1 (1.2, 3.6) 4.0 (2.6–6.1)	Daily dose No use Ibuprofen≤1500mg Ibuprofen>1500mg Naproxen≤750mg Naproxen>750mg Diclofenac≤100mg Diclofenac>100mg Indomethacin≤75mg Indomethacin>75mg	RR UGIB (95% CI) 1.0 2.1 (1.1, 4.1) 6.5 (2.6, 16.4) 4.0 (1.3, 11.8) 3.1 (1.4, 6.6) 4.1 (2.7, 7.6) 3.4 (1.4, 8.5) 1.4 (0.3, 5.8) 14.4 (5.7, 36.4)
	RR increases by 12% (9%,15%) for every unit increase in the dose taken in the previous week.			
Timing of exposure	Current users ≤4 weeks Current users >4 weeks Recent past users	OR (95% CI) 6.3 (3.5, 11.3) 2.5 (2.0, 3.3) 0.9 (0.65, 1.3)	Bleeding only RR (95% CI) Current use 3.9 (3.1, 4.9) Recent use 1.9 (1.3, 2.9) Past use 1.2 (0.8, 1.6)	Perforation RR (95% CI) 7.9 (5.7, 10.9) 2.1 (1.0, 4.4) 1.9 (1.1, 3.3)

UGIB=upper GI bleeding; RR=relative risk; OR=odds ratio; GI=gastrointestinal. [a]Small of standard dose units consumed in the previous week. [c]Cut-off daily doses for low, medium and indomethacin <75 mg, 75–149 mg, ≥150 mg; ibuprofen <1200 mg, 1200–1799 mg, ≥1800 ≥1000 mg; piroxicam <10 mg, 20 mg, ≥30 mg. [d]Doses as defined in data sheets.

Langman et al. 1994[3]		MacDonald et al. 1997[4]	
Peptic ulcer bleeding[a]		UGIB, perforation[a]	
Population-based, case-control study *n* = 1144 cases, 2115 controls		Population-based, (>50 years) case-control study *n* = 52,293 cases, 73,792 controls	
During last 3 m	OR (95% CI)		UGIB/perforation RR (95% CI)
No use	1.0		
Ibuprofen	2.0 (1.4, 2.8)	Fenbufen	0.4 (0.1, 1.9)
Diclofenac	4.2 (2.6, 6.8)	Nabumetone	0.6 (0.1, 2.7)
Any NA-NSAID	4.5 (3.6, 5.6)	Indomethacin	1.0 (0.4, 2.3)
Naproxen	9.1 (5.5, 15.1)	Ibuprofen	1.0
Indomethacin	11.3 (6.3, 20.3)	Mefenamic acid	1.4 (0.7, 2.8)
Piroxicam	13.7 (7.1, 26.3)	Diclofenac	1.4 (0.6, 3.1)
Ketoprofen	23.7 (7.6, 74.2)	Naproxen	1.4 (0.8, 2.5)
Azapropazone	31.5 (10.3, 96.9)	Ketoprofen	1.4 (0.6, 3.4)
		Piroxicam	3.3 (1.9, 5.8)
		Azapropazone	3.7 (1.9, 7.4)
Dose within[c] past month	OR (95% CI)		UGIB/perforation RR (95% CI)
		Low[d]	1.0
No use	1.0	Medium[d]	1.4 (1.0, 1.9)
Low	2.5 (1.7, 3.8)	High[d]	1.9 (1.2, 3.1)
Medium	4.5 (3.3, 6.0)		
High	8.6 (5.8, 12.6)		
	OR (95% CI)	UGIB/perforation	
Single/multiple NSAIDs in past month ±previous use	4.8 (3.8–6.0)		RR (95% CI)
		No NSAID exposure	1.0
NSAIDs in past month & duration		Current NSAID	
≥3 m	3.8 (2.9, 5.1)		8.0 (5.6, 11.4)
Single NSAID taken in past month ±previous use	4.4 (3.4, 5.5)	Year post-exposure	
NSAID started in past month	9.6 (5.5, 16.8)		3.0 (2.1, 4.3)
		Constant risk during continuous exposure, excess risk for 1 year post-exposure	

numbers in each case had perforation, but were not separated from the total. [b]Number and high dose categories: azapropazone <600 mg, 600–899 mg, ≥900 mg; diclofenac mg; ketoprofen <100 mg, 100–199 mg, ≥200 mg; naproxen <500 mg, 500–999 mg,

Table 2 Risks of acute and chronic renal failure associated with the use of NSAIDs

	Sandler et al. 1991[5]		Evans et al. 1995[6]	
Outcomes	Risk for chronic renal disease associated with NSAID use		Risk for acute renal failure with NSAID and aspirin use	
Type of study	Population-based, case-control study 554 cases, 516 controls		Population-based, case-control study 207 cases, 1238 community controls 411 hospital controls	
Estimated RR/OR	Men: use frequency	OR (95% CI) Adj[a]	Community controls	OR (95% CI) Unadj[b]
	Never	1.0	Oral NSAIDs	
	Occasional	1.9 (0.7, 4.9)	Recent exposure	2.2 (1.5, 3.3)
	Weekly	0.8 (0.2, 3.0)	Previous	1.5 (1.1, 2.1)
	Daily	4.6 (1.5, 14.0)	Topical NSAIDs	
	Men: use duration		Recent exposure	1.3 (0.5, 3.9)
	<2 years	4.2 (0.5, 37.7)	Previous	1.8 (1.1, 2.9)
	2–4 years	4.5 (0.5, 41.5)	Aspirin	
	≥5 years	4.8 (1.1, 23.1)	Recent exposure	1.7 (1.0, 2.9)
			Previous	2.1 (1.4, 3.2)
	Women: use frequency			
	Never	1.0	**Hospital controls**	
	Occasional	0.6 (0.2, 1.5)	Oral NSAIDs	
	Weekly	1.8 (0.6, 5.6)	Recent exposure	1.8 (1.2, 2.9)
	Daily	1.1 (0.4, 2.7)	Previous	1.1 (0.8, 1.5)
	Women: use duration		Topical NSAIDs	
	<2 years	2.9 (0.3, 26.5)	Recent exposure	0.6 (0.2, 1.4)
	2–4 years	0.7 (0.8, 2.8)	Previous	1.2 (0.7, 2.0)
	≥5 years	1.0 (0.2, 5.0)	Aspirin	
			Recent exposure	0.8 (0.5, 1.3)
			Previous	0.9 (0.6, 1.4)

RR=relative risk; OR=odds ratio. [a]Adj=adjusted for matching factors and income; OR analyses were calculated for recent exposure to oral NSAIDs and previous exposure to single logistic regression model including terms for the variables listed; cardiovascular heart failure, myocardial ischaemia, or arrythmia during the 5 months prior to the index

BACKGROUND

NSAIDs have been repeatedly shown to be important causes of major GI bleeding and ulcer perforation. The estimates of risk summarized in Table 1 are from a selection of recently published case-control studies[1-4]. It should be noted that randomized trials, because of their small size and short duration, have provided relatively little information on risk with 'classical' NSAIDs. Although evidence from non-randomized, observational studies is generally ranked poorly in

Perez Gutthann et al. 1996[7]	Henry et al. 1997[8]
Risk for acute renal failure with NSAID use	Risk for functional renal impairment associated with NSAID use in the elderly
Population-based, retrospective case-control study 306 cases, 1997 controls	Population-based, case-control study 110 cases, 189 controls

Use frequency	OR (95% CI) Adj[c]	Use frequency	OR (95% CI) Adj[d]
Never	1.0	Past month	2.0 (0.98, 3.9)
Current	4.1 (1.5, 10.8)	Past week	1.5 (0.8, 2.8)
Recent	0.8 (0.2, 4.1)		
Past	1.5 (0.4, 5.6)		
		History No renal disease, no gout/ hyperuricaemia	
Current users' dose/duration of use			
No use	1.0		0.6 (0.2, 1.6)
Low dose	4.0 (1.1, 15.2)	+ renal disease, no gout/ hyperuricaemia	
High dose	9.8 (3.2, 30.5)		
≤1 month	8.5 (2.5, 28.6)		6.6 (0.8, 57.9)
2–6 months	3.2 (0.8, 13.0)	No renal disease, + gout/ hyperuricaemia	
>6 months	2.7 (0.7, 9.9)		
			71 (1.3, 39.7)
Males	1.0	+ renal disease, + gout/ hyperuricaemia	
Females	0.6 (0.3, 1.4)		
			82.2 (4.1, 1661.1)
15–64 years	1.0		
65+	3.5 (1.3, 9.8)		
Cardiovascular risk indicator			
No	1.0		
Yes	2.7 (1.0, 7.3)		

compares users with non-users. [b]Unadj=unadjusted. Adjusted conditional logistic regression topical NSAIDs and aspirin, but differed little from the unadjusted. [c]OR calculated from a risk indicator was defined as the use of drugs with indications for hypertension, congestive date. [d]NSAID ORs adjusted for age, history of heart disease, history of renal disease.

evidence-based medicine, the data relating to NSAIDs are strong. As can be seen in Table 1, the relative risk estimates are high, and consistent; dose–response relationships have been shown repeatedly, the effects of timing of therapy have been well investigated and patients with particular susceptibilities have been identified. In addition, there is a good biological basis for the damage caused by these drugs.

In comparison to GI effects, the impact of NSAIDs on the kidney has been less well investigated. The main impact of treatment is functional renal impairment,

Table 3 *Comparative GI toxicity of individual NSAIDs and their comparative COX-2/COX-1 ratios higher ratios indicate more potent inhibition of COX-1*

Drug	Henry et al. 1996[9] GI toxicity: summary ranking method. Mean rank (S.D.)[a]	Akarasereenont et al.[12] COX-2/COX-1 ratio (intact cells)[b]	Vane and Botting 1996[13] COX-2/COX-1 ratio (intact cells)[b]
Ibuprofen	1.0	15	15
Diclofenac	2.3 (0.5)	0.7	0.7
Fenoprofen	3.5 (1.2)	–	–
Diflunisal	3.5 (0.5)	–	–
Sulindac	6.0 (0)	102	100
Naproxen	7.0 (0)	0.6	0.6
Indomethacin	8.0 (0)	57	60
Piroxicam	9.0 (0)	300	250
Ketoprofen	10.3 (0.5)	–	–
Tolmetin	11.0 (0.9)	176	175
Azapropazone	11.7 (0.5)	–	–

IC_{50}=concentration at which 50% activity is inhibited; BAEC=bovine aortic endothelial lowest relative risk. [b]COX-1 from whole cell cultures of BAEC; COX-2 from whole cell [c]Stimulation with bacterial endotoxin.

which is ischaemic in aetiology. Affected patients, by virtue of volume depletion, or co-existing disease, have high circulating levels of noradrenaline and angiotensin II, and rely on renal prostaglandin production to maintain renal blood flow[11]. In the presence of an NSAID, renal ischaemia develops and glomerular filtration drops. NSAIDs have also been associated with interstitial nephritis and other forms of renal damage. Renal outcomes have been investigated in a small number of epidemiological studies, four of which are summarized in Table 2[5-8]. It can be seen that the studies have tended to concentrate on kidney disease rather than functional renal impairment as the outcome. However, they are consistent in showing a moderate risk associated with the use of classical NSAIDs.

in different systems; IC_{50} of indomethacin for COX-1 and COX-2 across a range of systems –

COX-2/COX-1 ratio (system)	Jouzeau et al. 1997[16] Indomethacin IC_{50} mol/l System	COX-1	COX-2
	Purified animal		
3.1 (transfected cos-1 cells)[14]	Seminal vesicle	$0.2–0.6\times10^{-6}$	–
2.2 (guinea pig macrophages)[15]	Sheep placenta	–	$4.1–15\times10^{-6}$
–	**Recombinant murine** homogenate	$10–200\times10^{-9}$	$50–300\times10^{-9}$
–			
	Recombinant human		
39 (transfected cos-1 cells)[14]	Sf9 purified	$0.1–1.7\times10^{-6}$	$0.4–25\times10^{-6}$
–	Sf21 homogenate	0.1×10^{-6}	0.9×10^{-6}
	Whole cells: animal		
30 (guinea pig macrophages)[15]	Guinea pig macrophages	0.2×10^{-9}	–
33 (guinea pig macrophages)[15]	Guinea pig macrophages		
–	+ LPSc	–	6.4×10^{-9}
–	RAEC	0.03×10^{-6}	–
–	J774.2 + LPSc	–	1.7×10^{-6}
–	**Whole cells: human** U937	$5–20\times10^{-9}$	–
	Osteosarcoma 143	–	$10–50\times10^{-9}$
	COS cells (rhCOX)	20×10^{-9}	30×10^{-9}
	Platelets	3.2×10^{-8}	–
	Monocytes + LPSc	–	1.6×10^{-9}
	Whole blood	0.2×10^{-6}	0.5×10^{-6}

cells; Rh=recombinant human; GI=gastrointestinal. [a]Lowest rank score is equivalent to cultures of murine J774.2 macrophages stimulated with lipopolysaccharide (LPS).

RELATIONSHIP OF EPIDEMIOLOGICAL RISKS TO COX-2 SELECTIVITY

Most available information relates to the GI side effects of NSAIDs. With a group of colleagues, including many of the original investigators, we were able to pool the results of high quality epidemiological studies of the risk of major GI complications of therapy[9]. The large size of the data set enabled us to assess and then rank the relative risk of major GI bleeding with individual NSAIDs. Summary ranking data are given in Table 3 for those drugs in relation to their COX-2 selectivity. COX-2/COX-1 ratios are listed for most of the drugs and are based on work using intact cell systems[12,13]. We recognize that there has been considerable controversy over the best assay system for measuring COX-2 selectivity. COX-2/COX-1 ratios vary according to the system used[12–16]. The variability between systems is illustrated by the range of IC_{50} values obtained for indomethacin against both COX isoenzymes using different enzyme and cell systems[16]. However, as can be seen, and has been pointed out previously, there is an apparent inverse correlation between the magnitude of the relative risk of major GI complications and the degree of COX-2 selectivity. This is what is anticipated from the results of experimental studies.

Some caveats have to be stated. In compiling the data in Table 3, neither dosage nor drug half life has been considered as confounders of the epidemiological estimates of risk. We have previously shown that the rank order of GI toxicity also correlates with drug half-life, being higher in drugs with a long plasma half life (Table 4)[1]. Epidemiological studies have shown a linear dose-response relationship between the magnitude of the relative risk of GI bleeding and an estimate of the 'standardized' doses of NSAIDs that have been consumed in the previous week or month (Table 1). In Table 5, it can be seen that, to some degree, drugs with low COX-2 selectivity (high COX-2/COX-1 ratio) tend to have longer half lives than those with a high degree of COX-2 selectivity. To adjust for these potential confounders by multivariate analysis is difficult as the systematic review we performed was not based on data from individual subjects. Instead, we pooled across studies, and across drugs, and the number of drugs for which complete data are available is too small to enable the appropriate adjustments to be carried out. Nevertheless, visual inspection of the data indicates that some degree of confounding is likely, and may explain in part the apparent correlation between the degree of COX-2 selectivity and the magnitude of relative risk.

In general, the studies of renal failure provide insufficient data to assess the role of COX-2 selectivity. The studies have not been large enough to assess the level of risk with individual NSAIDs and the study endpoints have been diverse. In our case-control study of functional renal impairment, we have been able to look at the independent effects of COX-2 selectivity, drug half life and ingested dose on the level of risk for this outcome (Table 6). In this case, we have used the individual patient data. In a univariate analysis, the relative risk of renal impairment increased across strata defined by the ratios of COX-2/COX-1. Aspirin has been excluded from this table as it was used in very low prophylactic doses, at which it would not be expected to have an effect on renal function. The univariate analysis suggests a relationship, and in column three this relationship holds after adjustment for ingested dose. However, in column four, the analysis is simultaneously adjusted for the published value for the plasma half life of the individual drugs, and the relationship between risk and COX-2/COX-1 ratio disappears. This does not mean that COX-2 selectivity is unimportant, but indicates that the apparent association in the univariate analysis may be confounded by drug half life.

Table 4 Comparison of ranking of individual NSAIDs by relative risk of GI complications and plasma half life

Comparator	GI toxicity: rank by relative risk, lowest to highest	Plasma half lives (h)		
		Main analysis	Sensitivity analysis I	Sensitivity analysis II
Ibuprofen	1	2.0	2.0	2.0
Diclofenac	2	1.5	1.5	1.5
Diflunisal	3	10.8	10.8	10.8
Fenoprofen	4	2.2	2.2	2.2
Aspirin	5	0.5	4.5	4.5
Sulindac	6	7.8	7.8	16.4
Naproxen	7	14.0	14.0	14.0
Indomethacin	8	3.8	3.8	3.8
Piroxicam	9	48.0	48.0	48.0
Ketoprofen	10	2.0	8.5	8.5
Tolmetin	11	6.8	6.8	6.8
Azapropazone	12	22.0	22.0	22.0
Rank correlation Kendall's tau		0.3692	0.5038	0.4733
(P value)		(0.0947)	(0.0226)	(0.0322)

Main analysis used $t_{1/2}$ for aspirin (not salicylic acid) and for ketoprofen in its conventional formulation. Sensitivity analysis I used $t_{1/2}$ for salicylic acid and for the sustained release formulation of ketoprofen. Sensitivity analysis II substituted the $t_{1/2}$ for the sulphide metabolite of sulindac for that of the parent drug and was otherwise the same as sensitivity analysis I. Source Henry et al. 1998[17].

Table 5 Estimated relative risks of upper GI complications associated with the use of individual NSAIDs

Drug	Odds ratio (95% CI)[1]	Average dose[a] consumed by NSAID-using case patients	Half life (h)	COX-2/COX-1 ratio[12]	COX-2/COX-1 ratio[13]	COX-2/COX-1 ratio (system)
Ibuprofen	0.7 (0.4, 2.4)	6.5	2	15	15	3.1 (transfected cos-1 cells)[14]
Diflunisal	1.0 (0.4, 2.4)	11.3	8–12	–	–	–
Diclofenac	1.7 (1.1, 2.5)	7.7	1–2	0.7	0.7	2.2 (guinea pig macrophages)[15]
Sulindac	2.1 (1.1, 4.1)	11.2	7	102	100	39 (transfected cos-1 cells)[14]
Indomethacin	2.5 (1.5, 4.1)	6.3	3	57	60	30 (guinea pig macrophages)[15]
Naproxen	2.8 (1.8, 4.3)	5.5	14	0.6	0.6	–
Ketoprofen (sustained release)	3.6 (2.0, 6.6)	11.9	8	–	–	–
Piroxicam	4.8 (2.6, 8.7)	4.7	50	300	250	33 (guinea pig macrophages)[15]

GI=gastrointestinal. [a]Number of standard doses consumed in the week before the index day.

Table 6 Odds ratios (OR), stratified by COX-1/COX-2 ratios, for functional renal impairment based on univariate, multi-variate and multi-variate + $t_{1/2}$ analyses of individual patient data. Reanalysis of data from Henry et al. 1997[8].

COX-2/COX-1- ratio	Univariate OR (95% CI)[a]	Multivariate OR (95% CI)[b]	Multivariate and $T_{1/2}$ OR (95% CI)[c]
No NSAID	1	1	1
≤0.7	2.1 (0.8, 5.2)	2.1 (0.8, 6.1)	1.0 (0.3, 3.8)
15–100	3.7 (1.2, 11.2)	2.5 (0.7, 9.0)	2.3 (0.6, 8.7)
600	12.0 (1.3, 114.3)	7.1 (0.6, 89.4)	0.1 (0.001, 8.4)

[a]Univariate ORs were calculated using conditional logistic regression (matched on age within five years and sex). Test for log linear trend, $P=0.023$. [b]Multivariate ORs adjusted for age in years, a history of gout, a past history of heart disease, a past history of renal disease and ingested dose. Test for log linear trend, $P=0.033$. [c]These ORs are adjusted as for [b], and in addition, for $t_{1/2}$. Test for log linear trend, P not significant.

CONCLUSIONS

We believe that COX-2 selectivity will prove to be important, and anticipate that drugs which are selective for this isoform of COX will be safer in clinical practice. This is crucially important from a public health standpoint, in view of the extent of use of anti-inflammatory drugs in most communities. Consequently, the evidence on which we base future prescribing decisions should be of high quality. Large epidemiological studies conducted with the newer NSAIDs may show improved safety, but we believe that there is a need for large randomized trials with clinical endpoints. The data on the effects of the classical NSAIDs are interesting, but we believe that they are not particularly informative in respect of COX selectivity. The existing data are open to different interpretations, and at least some of the effects can be explained by factors such as ingested dose or plasma half life. Because the issue is so important, we do not believe that arguments should be centred on the interpretation of these data, but instead should be based on the results of large, high-quality, randomized, controlled trials of new agents, using clinically meaningful endpoints.

REFERENCES

1. Henry D, Dobson A, Turner C. Variability in the risk of major gastrointestinal complications from nonaspirin nonsteroidal anti-inflammatory drugs. *Gastroenterology*. 1993;105:1078–88.
2. Garcia Rodriguez LA, Alberto L, Jick H. Risk of upper gastro-intestinal bleeding and perforation associated with individual non-steroidal anti-inflammatory drugs. *Lancet*. 1994;343:769–72.
3. Langman MJS, Weil J, Wainwright P, Lawson DH, Rawlins MD, Logan RFA et al. Risks of bleeding peptic ulcer associated with individual non-steroidal anti-inflammatory drugs. *Lancet*. 1994;343:1075–8.

4. MacDonald TM, Morant SV, Robinson GC, Shield MJ, McGilchrist MM, Murray FE et al. Association of upper gastrointestinal toxicity of non-steroidal anti-inflammatory drugs with continued exposure: cohort study. *Br Med J*. 1997;315:1333–7.

5. Sandler DP, Burr R, Weinberg CR. Nonsteroidal anti-inflammatory drugs and the risk for chronic renal disease. *Ann Intern Med*. 1991;115:165–72.

6. Evans JMM, McGregor E, McMahon AD, McGilchrist MM, Jones MC, White G et al. Non-steroidal anti-inflammatory drugs and hospitalisation for acute renal failure. *Q J Med*. 1995;88:551–7.

7. Perez Gutthann S, Garcia Rodriguez LA, Raiford DS, Duque Oliart A, Ris Romeu J. Non-steroidal anti-inflammatory drugs and the risk of hospitalisation for acute renal failure. *Arch Intern Med*. 1996;156:2433–9.

8. Henry D, Page J, Whyte I, Nanra R, Hall C. Consumption of non-steroidal anti-inflammatory drugs and the development of functional renal impairment in elderly subjects. Results of a case-control study. *Br J Clin Pharmacol*. 1997;44:85–90.

9. Henry D, L-Y Lim L, Garcia Rodriguez LA, Perez Gutthann S, Carson JL, Griffin M et al. Variability in risk for gastrointestinal complications with individual non-steroidal anti-inflammatory drugs: results of a collaborative meta-analysis. *Br Med J*. 1996;312:1563–6.

10. Vane JR. NSAIDs, COX-2 inhibitors and the gut. *Lancet*. 1995;346:1105–6.

11. Clive DM, Stoff JS. Renal syndromes associated with non-steroidal anti-inflammatory drugs. *N Engl J Med*. 1984;310:563–72.

12. Akarasereenont P, Kongpatanakul S, Henry DA, Thiemermann C. The side effects of non-steroidal anti-inflammatory drugs: are they attributed to the selective inhibition of different isoforms of cyclo-oxygenase? *Siriraj Hosp Gaz*. 1997;49:1172–7.

13. Vane JR, Botting RM. Mechanism of action of anti-inflammatory drugs. *Scand J Rheumatol*. 1996;25(suppl 102):9–21.

14. Laneuville O, Breuer DK, DeWitt DL, Hla T, Funk CD, Smith WL. Differential inhibition of human prostaglandin endoperoxide H synthases-1 and -2 by non-steroidal anti-inflammatory drugs. *J Pharmacol Exp Ther*. 1994;271:927–37.

15. Furst DE. Meloxicam: selective COX-2 inhibition in clinical practice. *Semin Arthritis Rheum*. 1997;26:21–7.

16. Jouzeau J-Y, Terlain B, Abid A, Nedelec E, Netter P. Cyclo-oxygenase isoenzymes. How recent findings affect thinking about nonsteroidal anti-inflammatory drugs. *Drugs*. 1997;53:563–82.

17. Henry D, Drew A, Beuzeville S. Adverse drug reactions in the gastrointestinal system attributed to ibuprofen. In: Rainsford KD, Powanda MC editors. *Safety and Efficacy of Non-prescription (OTC) Analgesics and NSAIDs*. Dordrecht; The Netherlands: Kluwer Academic Publishers; 1998:19–45.

16

Overview of MELISSA and SELECT clinical trials of meloxicam

A. KAHAN

Classical non-steroidal anti-inflammatory drugs (NSAIDs) provide effective treatment for rheumatic disease, but their use may be limited by gastrointestinal (GI) side effects. The most common side effects such as dyspepsia, abdominal pain and nausea are not serious, but may result in decreased patient compliance or discontinuation of treatment. However, the serious NSAID-related GI side effects of perforations, ulcerations and bleeding (PUBs) are estimated to be responsible for 0.13% of patient deaths per year[1]; a significant healthcare problem considering the number of prescriptions for NSAIDs. There is, therefore, a need for new NSAIDs with improved GI tolerability.

The discovery of two isoforms of cyclooxygenase (COX)[2] led to the hypothesis that inhibition of the inducible isoform, COX-2, was responsible for the anti-inflammatory effect of classical NSAIDs, whilst inhibition of the constitutively expressed COX-1 isoform was responsible for their GI toxicity[3].

Meloxicam is one of the first clinically available selective COX-2 inhibitors[4]. The preferential inhibition of COX-2 relative to COX-1 by meloxicam has been demonstrated in a number of in vitro, ex vivo and in vivo systems, whereas diclofenac, piroxicam, indomethacin and naproxen either inhibited both COX isoforms to a similar extent or preferentially inhibited COX-1[5-8].

Double-blind trials in over 5000 patients with either osteoarthritis (OA) or rheumatoid arthritis have shown that meloxicam has an improved GI tolerability compared with equi-effective doses of the classical NSAIDs, piroxicam (20 mg), naproxen (750 to 1000 mg) and diclofenac (100 mg slow release [SR])[9]. The Meloxicam Large-scale International Study Safety Assessment (MELISSA)[10] and the Safety and Efficacy Large-scale Evaluation of COX-inhibiting Therapies (SELECT)[11] trials have further investigated the tolerability of once-daily treatment with meloxicam 7.5 mg, compared with diclofenac 100 mg SR (MELISSA) or piroxicam 20 mg (SELECT) for 28 days, in 17,979 patients with acute exacerbation of OA of the knee, hip, hand or spine.

METHODS

The design, patient selection, methods and study protocols of the MELISSA and SELECT studies were identical except for the selection of the comparator, either diclofenac 100 mg SR in the MELISSA study or piroxicam 20 mg in the SELECT study. The methods have been described elsewhere[10,11] and so they will only be outlined briefly here.

Design and Patients

These were prospective, international, large-scale, double-blind, double-dummy, randomized trials. Most patients were recruited from general practice and were eligible if they: were aged at least 18 years; suffered from acute and painful exacerbation of OA of the knee, hip, hand or spine; had pain on active movement exceeding 35 mm on a 100 mm visual analogue scale (VAS) (where 0 mm = no pain and 100 mm = unbearable pain); and were considered suitable for treatment with an NSAID. Exclusion criteria were chosen to reflect prescribing recommendations for meloxicam and to exclude conditions which could interfere with evaluation of the treatments.

Treatment and Assessments

After a wash-out period of three days for previously taken NSAIDs, patients were randomized for daily treatment with meloxicam 7.5 mg, diclofenac 100 mg SR (MELISSA patients were randomized 1:1 to meloxicam or diclofenac), or piroxicam 20 mg (SELECT patients were randomized 1:1 to meloxicam or piroxicam) for 28 days.

Tolerability of the treatments was determined by: the incidence, severity and relationship to treatment of adverse events (assessed at baseline and endpoint), particularly GI adverse events; withdrawals due to adverse events; and final global tolerability assessed by the patient and physician on a 4-point verbal rating scale (VRS) (1 = good, 2 = satisfactory, 3 = not satisfactory, 4 = bad). PUBs of the upper GI tract were assessed; the presence of ulceration or bleeding was confirmed by endoscopy, and the presence of perforation was confirmed by endoscopy, surgery, or X-ray. Patients reporting melaena were also regarded as having PUBs even if no endoscopy was performed or clinical evidence of bleeding was given.

Efficacy endpoints were assessed at baseline and at the end of the treatment period or at the point of treatment withdrawal. Assessments for efficacy included: pain on active movement and at rest on a 100 mm VAS; global efficacy assessment and global assessment by patient and physician on a 4-point VRS; patient assessment of arthritic condition on the same 4-point VRS; patient assessment of change in arthritic condition and change in patient status on a 3-point VRS

(1 = improved, 2 = unchanged, 3 = deteriorated); and withdrawals due to lack of efficacy.

Statistical Analysis

An intention-to-treat analysis was performed using the last value carried forward for efficacy parameters in patients who withdrew before the end of the trial. The odds ratios between treatment groups were calculated for adverse events and GI adverse events and were analysed with Fisher's exact test. Clinically significant differences in efficacy were calculated prior to the start of the study using the consensus guidelines for OA clinical trials[12] based on criteria previously identified by the Food and Drug Administration and European League Against Rheumatism as important outcomes for OA clinical trials. Minimum clinically significant differences were: 17.5 mm and 10.5 mm on a VAS for pain on active movement and pain at rest, respectively; 0.8 (VRS) for global efficacy; 0.67 (VRS) for patient status; and 0.8 (VRS) for arthritic condition. In order to determine whether the differences between treatment groups reached one-half of these pre-defined minimum clinically significant differences, t-tests were performed and 95% confidence intervals for the mean differences between treatment groups were calculated.

RESULTS

A total of 19,337 patients were enrolled and randomized to treatment; 1358 of these did not receive treatment due to violations of entry criteria. Thus, 17,979 patients who received treatment were evaluated on an intention-to-treat basis for safety and efficacy; a total of 8955 patients received meloxicam 7.5 mg once-daily (4635 in the MELISSA study and 4320 in the SELECT study), 4688 received diclofenac 100 mg SR once-daily, and 4336 received piroxicam 20 mg once-daily. In the MELISSA study, significantly more of the patients who received meloxicam completed the study protocol compared with diclofenac-treated patients (90% vs 88%, P=0.0014). In the SELECT study, 89% and 88% in the meloxicam and piroxicam groups, respectively, completed the trial.

Demographic and baseline disease characteristics were comparable between the patient groups (Table 1). Approximately 40% of the study population were aged over 65 years.

Tolerability

Significantly fewer patients receiving treatment with meloxicam experienced adverse events than patients treated with the comparator drug, diclofenac (27% vs 32%, P<0.001) or piroxicam (23% vs 28%, P<0.001) (Table 2). This difference was largely due to the lower incidence of GI adverse events in the meloxicam groups compared with the diclofenac group (13% vs 19%, P<0.001) and the piroxicam group (10% vs 15%, P<0.001).

Dyspepsia, abdominal pain, nausea and vomiting, and diarrhoea were the most commonly reported GI adverse events and occurred less frequently with

Table 1 Demographic and baseline characteristics of patients

	MELISSA		SELECT	
	Meloxicam 7.5 mg (n = 4635)	Diclofenac 100 mg SR (n = 4688)	Meloxicam 7.5 mg (n = 4320)	Piroxicam 20 mg (n = 4336)
Male:female (%)	33:67	33:67	32:68	33:67
Mean age in years (S.D.)	61.5 (12.7)	61.7 (12.5)	61.3 (12.3)	61.6 (12.3)
≤65 years (%)	60	59	63	61
>65 years (%)	40	41	37	39
Location of OA (%)				
Hand	12	12	12	11
Hip	15	17	14	15
Knee	45	41	46	44
Spine	28	30	28	30
Median duration of OA (months)	52	48	45	48
History of PUBs (%)	4.8	5.3	6.4	5.6
Concomitant administration of drugs for gastroprotection during the trial (%)	5.6	6.4	4.6	5.6
Previous use of NSAIDS (%)	82	82	79	79

Table 2 Overview of adverse events (AEs)

	MELISSA		SELECT	
Patients (%)	Meloxicam 7.5 mg (n = 4635)	Diclofenac 100 mg SR (n = 4688)	Meloxicam 7.5 mg (n = 4320)	Piroxicam 20 mg (n = 4336)
Any AE	27	32[a]	23	28[a]
GI AE	13	19[a]	10	15[a]
Withdrawn due to AE	5.5	8.0[a]	6.1	7.2[b]
Withdrawn due to GI AE	3.0	6.1[a]	3.8	5.3[c]

[a]$P<0.001$; [b]$P=0.0546$; [c]$P=0.0012$

meloxicam than with diclofenac or piroxicam ($P<0.05$) (Figure 1), with the exception of diarrhoea in the piroxicam group, where significance was not reached.

Significantly fewer patients treated with meloxicam withdrew from the study due to adverse events compared with those treated with diclofenac

Figure 1 Comparison of GI adverse events with meloxicam, diclofenac and piroxicam

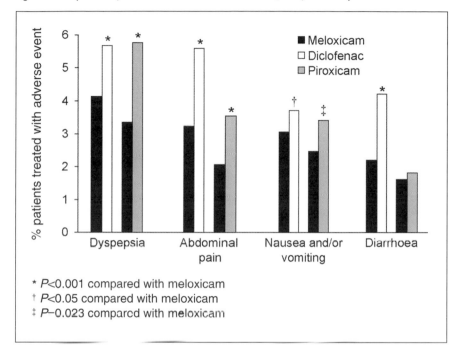

* *P*<0.001 compared with meloxicam
† *P*<0.05 compared with meloxicam
‡ *P*=0.023 compared with meloxicam

(5.5% vs 8.0%, *P*<0.001) (Table 2). This difference was largely accounted for by the decreased number of withdrawals due to GI adverse events with meloxicam compared with diclofenac (3.0% vs 6.1%, *P*<0.001). Similarly, fewer patients treated with meloxicam withdrew due to adverse events compared with those receiving piroxicam treatment, but this difference did not reach statistical significance (6.1% vs 7.2%, *P*=0.0546). However, significantly fewer patients treated with meloxicam withdrew due to GI adverse events than those treated with piroxicam (3.8% vs 5.3%, *P*=0.0012).

Serious adverse events occurred in 56 and 52 patients in the meloxicam and diclofenac groups of the MELISSA study, respectively, and in 26 and 30 patients in the meloxicam and piroxicam groups of the SELECT study, respectively. Less drug-related serious adverse events occurred in the meloxicam group than in the diclofenac group (13 vs 24).

A PUB was experienced by 0.13% of patients treated with meloxicam compared with 0.15% treated with diclofenac and 0.37% treated with piroxicam (Table 3). All of the eight confirmed ulcer complications, perforation or bleeding, occurred in the diclofenac or piroxicam groups.

There was a significant improvement in global tolerability assessed by patients or investigators with meloxicam compared with either diclofenac (*P*=0.0001 or *P*=0.0014 for patient and investigator ratings, respectively) or piroxicam (*P*<0.001 and *P*=0.002 for patient and investigator ratings, respectively).

Table 3 Patients with perforations, ulcerations or bleeding of the upper gastrointestinal tract

	MELISSA[a]		SELECT[b]	
	Meloxicam 7.5 mg (n = 4635)	Diclofenac 100 mg SR (n = 4688)	Meloxicam 7.5 mg (n = 4320)	Piroxicam 20 mg (n = 4336)
Duodenal ulcers				
Bleeding	0	1[c]	0	1
Perforated	0	2	0	0
Uncomplicated	1	0	0	1[d]
Gastric ulcers				
Bleeding	0	1	0	1
Perforated	0	0	0	2
Uncomplicated	1	2	2	4[e]
Haematemesis	1[f]	0	1[g]	1
Melaena	2[h]	1[i]	4	6[e]
Total	5	7	7	16

[a]Three patients who had an ulcer had a past history of PUB (one meloxicam, two diclofenac). [b]Five patients who had an ulcer had a past history of PUB (one meloxicam, four piroxicam). [c]Bleeding and perforated. [d]Not endoscopically verified. [e]One patient had concomitant duodenal ulcer. [f]Unclear whether haemotypsis or haematemesis. Endoscopy declined. No significant change in haemoglobin. [g]Patient suffered from concomitant duodenal ulcer and gastric ulcer. [h]Normal endoscopy in one, endoscopy declined in the second patient. No siginificant change in haemoglobin in either. [i]No significant change in haemoglobin. Endoscopy showed mild gastritis.

Pharmacoeconomic assessments were also favourable for meloxicam compared with both diclofenac and piroxicam. In the MELISSA study, three patients on meloxicam spent a total of five days in hospital because of GI adverse events compared with 10 patients on diclofenac who spent a total of 121 days in hospital for GI adverse events (includes one patient on diclofenac who stayed in hospital with both GI and other drug-related adverse events). Similarly, in the SELECT study, six patients in the meloxicam group and seven in the piroxicam group who were hospitalized for GI adverse events spent a total of 56 and 121 days, respectively, in hospital. Additionally, four patients on diclofenac and two on piroxicam spent a total of 31 and three days, respectively, in an intensive care unit (ICU) for GI adverse events. No patients on meloxicam were admitted to an ICU for GI adverse events.

Efficacy
Meloxicam, diclofenac and piroxicam gave equivalent improvements in pain on active movement and pain at rest (Figure 2), resulting in improvements in

Figure 2 Effect of treatment on pain on active movement and at rest measured on a 100 mm VAS (last observation carried forward; 95% confidence interval shown). The equivalence region indicates the pre-determined minimum clinically significant difference.

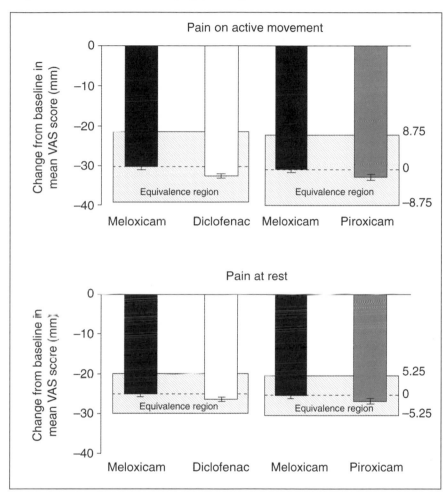

patient status, arthritic condition and a high assessment (by investigator and patient) of global efficacy (Table 4). Efficacy was equivalent for meloxicam, diclofenac and piroxicam treatment, according to the predefined equivalence boundaries[12]. Withdrawals due to lack of efficacy rarely occurred in the treatment groups. A similar proportion of patients withdrew prematurely due to lack of efficacy in the meloxicam and piroxicam groups of the SELECT study (1.7% vs 1.6%), but more patients withdrew due to lack of efficacy in the meloxicam group than in the diclofenac group of the MELISSA study (1.7% vs 1.0%, P<0.01).

Table 4 Summary of efficacy assessments

	MELISSA		SELECT	
	Meloxicam 7.5 mg	Diclofenac 100 mg SR	Meloxicam 7.5 mg	Piroxicam 20 mg
Pain on active movement (mm VAS); mean change from baseline (S.D.)	−30.3 (27.2)	−32.6 (26.4)	−31.0 (27.2)	−33.0 (27.2)
Pain at rest (mm VAS); mean change from baseline (S.D.)	−24.8 (28.1)	−26.3 (27.5)	−25.4 (28.5)	−26.9 (28.3)
Change in patient status[a]; mean (S.D.)	1.39 (0.58)	1.33 (0.55)	1.37 (0.57)	1.32 (0.54)
Arthritic condition[a]; mean change from baseline (S.D.)	−1.11 (1.07)	−1.21 (1.05)	−1.18 (1.07)	−1.25 (1.07)
Global efficacy assessed by the patient[b]; mean (S.D.)	1.98 (0.92)	1.85 (0.89)	1.93 (0.92)	1.86 (0.91)
Global efficacy assessed by the investigator[b]; mean (S.D.)	1.96 (0.88)	1.84 (0.85)	1.90 (0.88)	1.83 (0.87)

[a]Assessed on a 3-point verbal rating scale. [b]Assessed on a 4-point verbal rating scale.

DISCUSSION

Meloxicam demonstrated equivalent efficacy but improved GI tolerability compared with diclofenac and piroxicam in patients with OA, confirming the results of previous double-blind studies in over 5000 patients with OA and rheumatoid arthritis[9,13]. Improvements in pain on movement and pain at rest were comparable to those in a previous study in patients with OA[13] and resulted in improved ratings of patient status and arthritic condition, and a high assessment of global efficacy in all three treatment groups. Small differences in efficacy, in favour of diclofenac and piroxicam compared with meloxicam, did not reach the pre-determined levels of clinical significance. However, more patients treated with meloxicam discontinued due to lack of efficacy compared with those treated with diclofenac (P<0.01). These results suggest that differences in tolerability may have been partly due to differences in the effective dose; however, a careful interpretation is required. First, the differences between the two treatments were small compared with the pre-determined clinically significant difference. Furthermore, the significantly higher proportion of withdrawals in the diclofenac group compared with the meloxicam group (P=0.0014) would leave a higher number of patients receiving meloxicam treatment who could report lack of efficacy. Treatment failure is the direct result of patient withdrawal from therapy, irrespective of the reason for withdrawal. From this perspective, meloxicam treatment was comparable to piroxicam treatment but significantly better than diclofenac treatment. As significantly more meloxicam-treated patients successfully completed the study compared with diclofenac-treated patients one could postulate that effective long-term patient management would favour meloxicam over diclofenac.

These large-scale trials unequivocally demonstrate that once-daily treatment with meloxicam 7.5 mg results in improved GI tolerability compared with once-daily treatment with diclofenac 100 mg SR or piroxicam 20 mg. Meloxicam treatment resulted in significantly fewer GI adverse events compared with diclofenac (13% vs 19%, $P<0.001$) or piroxicam (10% vs 15%, $P<0.001$) treatment.

GI adverse events, such as PUBs, can be life-threatening and result in hospitalization[14]. Adverse events of the PUB category rarely occurred in patients treated with meloxicam (0.13%), diclofenac (0.15%) or piroxicam (0.37%). All eight confirmed cases of perforation or bleeding occurred in the diclofenac or piroxicam groups.

GI adverse events of mild severity, such as dyspepsia or nausea and vomiting, occurred significantly less frequently in the meloxicam treatment group than in the diclofenac or piroxicam groups. Although these adverse events are not life-threatening, they may cause a high level of patient discomfort and therefore influence patient compliance. Indeed, there were significantly fewer withdrawals due to GI adverse events in the meloxicam groups than in the diclofenac (3.0% vs 6.1%, $P<0.001$) or piroxicam (3.8% vs 5.3%, $P=0.0012$) groups.

Meloxicam was superior to diclofenac and piroxicam in pharmacoeconomic assessments, due to its improved GI tolerability. Meloxicam treatment resulted in fewer hospitalizations and a lower total number of patient days spent in hospital than diclofenac or piroxicam treatment. Additionally, four patients on diclofenac and two on piroxicam were admitted to an ICU ward with GI adverse events, but none of the patients treated with meloxicam. It has been estimated that treatment with meloxicam 7.5 mg once-daily would result in cost savings of 5% in Italy, 24% in the UK and 32% in France compared with once-daily diclofenac 100 mg SR, mainly due to savings in hospitalization costs[15].

CONCLUSIONS

These large-scale studies confirm the equivalent efficacy and superior tolerability of meloxicam 7.5 mg once-daily compared with equi-effective doses of the classical NSAIDs, diclofenac and piroxicam, in patients with symptomatic OA, supporting the concept that COX-2 inhibition underlies the efficacy of NSAIDs whilst some aspects of their toxicity are related to the inhibition of COX-1. In addition, data on treatment failures strongly suggest that prescribing NSAIDs with improved tolerance to patients with OA may result in more successful treatment outcomes. Long-term, intermittent, effective pain relief is essential in patients with OA as chronic pain syndromes lead to avoidance of activity and a vicious circle of inactivity, muscle weakness and joint instability. Mobilization of the patient with OA becomes a greater challenge to the clinician who is faced with a patient showing increasing signs of disability.

REFERENCES

1. Fries JF, Williams CA, Bloch DA, Michel BA. Nonsteroidal anti-inflammatory drug-associated gastropathy: incidence and risk factor models. *Am J Med*. 1991;91:213–22.
2. Masferrer JL, Seibert K, Zweifel B, Needleman P. Endogenous glucocorticoids regulate an inducible cyclo-oxygenase enzyme. *Proc Natl Acad Sci USA*. 1992;89:3917–21.
3. Vane J. Towards a better aspirin. *Nature*. 1994;367:215–6.
4. Degner F, Türck D, Pairet M. Pharmacological, pharmacokinetic and clinical profile of meloxicam. *Drugs Today*. 1997;33:739–58.
5. Mitchell JA, Akarasereenont P, Thiemerman C, Flower RJ, Vane JR. Selectivity of non-steroidal antiinflammatory drugs as inhibitors of constitutive and inducible cyclooxygenase. *Proc Natl Acad Sci USA*. 1993;90:11693–7.
6. Churchill L, Graham AG, Shih C-K, Pauletti D, Farina PR. Selective inhibition of human cyclo-oxygenase-2 by meloxicam. *Inflammopharmacology*. 1996;4:125–35.
7. Engelhardt G, Bögel R, Schnitzler C, Utzmann R. Meloxicam: influence on arachidonic acid metabolism. Part I. In vitro findings. *Biochem Pharmacol*. 1996;51:21–8.
8. Engelhardt G, Bögel R, Schnitzler C, Utzmann R. Meloxicam: influence on arachidonic acid metabolism. Part II. In vivo findings. *Biochem Pharmacol*. 1996;51:29–38.
9. Barner A. Review of clinical trials and benefit/risk ratio of meloxicam. *Scand J Rheumatol*. 1996;25(suppl 102):29–37.
10. Hawkey C, Kahan A, Steinbrück K, Alegre C, Baumelou E, Bégaud B et al. Gastrointestinal tolerability of meloxicam compared to diclofenac in osteoarthritis patients. *Br J Rheumatol*. 1998;37:937–45.
11. Dequeker J, Hawkey C, Kahan A, Alegre C, Baumelou E, Bégaud B et al. Improvement in gastrointestinal tolerability of the selective COX-2 inhibitor, meloxicam, compared with piroxicam: results of the Safety and Efficacy Large-scale Evaluation of COX-inhibiting Therapies (SELECT) trial in osteoarthritis. *Br J Rheumatol*. 1998;37:946–51.
12. Bellamy N, Carette S, Ford PM, Kean WF, le Riche NG, Lussier A. Osteoarthritis antirheumatic drug trials III. Setting the delta for clinical trials – results of a consensus development (Delphi) exercise. *J Rheumatol*. 1992;19:451–7.
13. Hosie J, Distel M, Bluhmki E. Meloxicam in osteoarthritis: a 6-month, double-blind comparison with diclofenac sodium. *Br J Rheumatol*. 1996;35(suppl 1):39–43.
14. Fries JF, Miller SR, Spitz W, Williams CA, Hubert HB, Bloch DA. Toward an epidemiology of gastropathy associated with nonsteroidal antiinflammatory drug use. *Gastroenterology*. 1989;96:647–55.
15. Jansen RB, Capri S, Nuijten MJC, Burrell A, Marini MG, Hardens M. Economic evaluation of meloxicam (7.5 mg) versus sustained release diclofenac (100 mg) treatment for osteoarthritis: a cross national assessment for France, Italy and the UK. *Br J Med Econ*. 1997;11:9–22.

The role of cyclooxygenase-2 in reproduction

P. BENNETT, R. SAWDY AND D. SLATER

Prostaglandins were originally discovered as the major constituents of seminal fluid that exhibited vasoactive properties[1]. They were originally thought to be a single substance secreted by the prostate gland and therefore termed 'prostaglandin' by Von Euler. In fact, seminal prostaglandins are a product of the seminal vesicles. It is possible that, had Von Euler known, we would now be talking about seminoglandins rather than prostaglandins. Prostaglandins are present in human seminal fluid in amounts approaching milligrams in each ejaculate. An association has been demonstrated between reduced prostaglandin levels and reduced male fertility[2], but beyond this, surprisingly little is known about the role of prostaglandins in seminal plasma. Prostaglandins have been found to be associated with ovarian function. Roles have been demonstrated or postulated in the initiation of follicular growth, in ovulation and in corpus luteum formation. Prostaglandins are formed predominantly in the granulosa cells of the preovulatory follicles and the highest concentrations are found at the time of ovulation. Cyclooxygenase (COX)-2 mRNA and protein are transiently induced by gonadotrophins in bovine granulosa cells of preovulatory follicles just prior to ovulation[3].

Prostaglandins also play a major role in blastocyst implantation. Increased uterine vascular permeability at sites of blastocyst apposition is one of the earliest events in the implantation process. This is preceded by generalized uterine oedema and luminal closure, and coincides with the initial attachment reaction between the trophectoderm and luminal epithelium[4]. Vasoactive prostaglandins have a role in these processes. Chakraborty et al.[5] found that the COX genes are differentially regulated in the peri-implantation mouse uterus. During the pre-implantation period COX-1 is expressed in the uterine epithelium until the initiation of the attachment reaction, after which expression is downregulated. This COX-1 expression coincides with the generalized uterine oedema required for luminal closure. The COX-2 gene is expressed in the luminal epithelium and subepithelial stromal cells at the antimesometrial pole exclusively surrounding the blastocyst at the time of the attachment reaction. They suggest that uterine COX-1 expression is influenced by ovarian steroids while the COX-2 gene is regulated by the implanting blastocyst during early pregnancy and that prostaglandins produced by COX-2 are involved in angiogenesis for the establishment of placentation. Drugs which block COX-2 may be effective in inhibition of ovulation and therefore as contraceptives, although the side effects of long-term blockage of COX-2 on other body systems are not yet known.

Although 90% of circulating prostaglandins are inactivated by one passage through the maternal pulmonary circulation, placental production of prostaglandins may lead to high circulating levels in the foetus, since blood flow through the foetal lung is less than 10% of cardiac output. Circulating prostaglandins maintain the patency of the ductus arteriosus, shunting blood from the right ventricle in the pulmonary trunk into the descending aorta. Following birth, increased oxygen tension within the ductus arteriosus causes a decrease in prostaglandin synthesis and duct closure is effected by the increased release of thromboxanes from the mature lung[6].

PROSTAGLANDIN-RELATED MOUSE KNOCKOUT EXPERIMENTS

Transgenic mice with knockouts for COX-1, COX-2 and the prostaglandin EP_4 and FP receptors have been reported[7–10]. Surprisingly, COX-1 knockout mice lack the gastrointestinal lesions that would be expected, given the importance of COX-1-mediated prostaglandin synthesis in the stomach. This may be because pharmacological inhibition of COX leaves intact the peroxidase activity. The only serious deficiency found in homozygous COX-1 knockout mice was their failure to produce viable offspring when homozygous mice were crossbred. Heterozygotes of either sex, when mated with homozygotes, produced litters of normal size and survival, indicating that COX-1 expression in only 50% of pups or their placentas is sufficient for the health of the entire litter. Breeding studies with COX-1 knock-out mice ruled out the need for COX-1 during ovulation or spermatogenesis, but suggested an essential requirement for COX-1 during mouse parturition.

The first report of a COX-2 knockout mouse, by Morham et al.[8], showed that homozygous COX-2 knockout mice begin to die at around eight weeks of age, with a few surviving for as long as 16 weeks. All tissues examined in these mice were normal except the kidney. Nephropathy was seen by six weeks in these animals, which increased in severity until death. Examination of COX-2-deleted mouse embryos showed that kidney maturation had ceased prematurely after only a small percentage of nephrons had developed, with the vast majority of glomeruli and tubules remaining small and immature. During postnatal life the small number of overworked functional nephrons begin to atrophy, with the development of glomerulosclerosis, interstitial inflammation and fibrosis, ultimately leading to kidney failure. In those mice which survived to adulthood, kidney lesions ranged from mild to severe with more severe lesions being more common in female than male homozygotes. This clearly shows an important role for COX-2 in the embryological development of the kidney. Fertility in COX-2 knockout mice was also dramatically reduced. Lim et al.[11] found that the number of ovulations is reduced in COX-2 knockout mice. Follicular development is normal in these mice but the administration of exogenous gonadotrophin did not restore the ovulation number. This finding is consistent with previous studies showing that gonadotrophins upregulate COX-2 during follicular development. Transfer of normal mouse blastocysts into COX-2 knockout recipients resulted in implantation failure, as did specific pharmacological inhibition of COX-2 in normal or heterozygous knockout animals, indicating a central role for COX-2 in mouse ovulation, implantation and decidualization.

Nguyen et al.[9] showed abnormal function of the ductus arteriosus in mice with deleted cyclic AMP-linked prostaglandin E receptor (EP_4). EP_4 receptor was found to be expressed in the smooth muscle of the mouse ductus arteriosus and homozygote deleted mice died in the postnatal period from failure of ductal closure. They suggested that the dependence of the ductus upon vasodilatory circulating prostaglandin F_2 during foetal life depends upon the presence of the EP_4 receptor. In the absence of EP_4 receptor expression the ductus does not become dependent and so remains patent after prostaglandin E_2 withdrawal at birth.

Sugimoto et al.[10] found that mice deleted for the prostaglandin FP receptor had normal oestrous cycles, normal ovulation and normal implantation. Pregnant homozygote FP knockout mice, however, failed to initiate labour because of failure of regression of the corpus luteum. In mice, the onset of labour is stimulated by regression of the corpus luteum and withdrawal of ovarian progesterone, which allows upregulation of the uterine oxytocin receptor. Ovariectomy in FP knockout homozygote mice released the progesterone inhibition allowing the onset of labour.

Whilst the respective roles of COX-1 and COX-2 in the menstrual cycle, ovulation and implantation may be similar in mice and humans, there appear to be fundamental differences both in the general mechanism of the onset of parturition and in the roles of COX-1 and -2 in parturition between the primate and the rodent. The corpus luteum regresses in the first trimester of human pregnancy and progesterone synthesis is taken over by the placenta and chorion. There is no large-scale withdrawal of progesterone in the human prior to parturition, although it has been suggested that there may be local withdrawal within the foetal membranes or changes in progesterone receptor function which leads to functional progesterone withdrawal. Although, in the mouse, COX-1-mediated prostaglandins appear to be important for normal parturition, in the human it is expression of COX-2 rather than COX-1 which increases within the uterus at term and it is doubtful whether COX-1 plays any significant role in the onset of human labour.

COX-2 IN HUMAN LABOUR

During pregnancy the uterus expands to accommodate the growing foetus and placenta, whilst remaining relatively quiescent, and the cervix remains firm and closed. Presumably 'pro-pregnancy' factors are in operation which inhibit myometrial contractility, but near to term 'pro-labour' factors predominate to mediate remodelling of the cervix to allow it to efface and dilate, and to stimulate coordinated uterine contractions. In sheep the onset of labour is associated with abrupt changes in foetal and maternal endocrine systems. Increased adrenocorticotrophic hormone (ACTH) release by the foetal anterior pituitary causes a progressive rise in foetal plasma glucocorticoid concentrations[12] which upregulates expression of the P450 17α-hydroxylase gene and so increases placental 17α-hydroxylase activity[13]. This causes an abrupt increase in maternal plasma oestrogen concentrations only a few days before the onset of labour. These abrupt changes are not seen in the human.

There is considerable evidence to support a central role for prostaglandins in sheep and in human parturition. Labour is associated with increased prostaglandin synthesis within the uterus[14] particularly from the foetal membranes[15]. Prostaglandins act to mediate cervical ripening and to stimulate uterine contractions[16] and indirectly to increase fundally-dominant myometrial contractility by upregulation of oxytocin receptors and synchronization of contractions[17,18].

Prostaglandins are formed from the precursor, arachidonic acid, which itself is a substrate for at least three enzyme groups. The COX, or prostaglandin endoperoxide synthase, pathway produces prostaglandins. The lipoxygenase enzyme pathways produce a series of hydroxyeicosatetraenoic acids (HETEs). Arachidonic acid metabolism via epoxygenase pathways produces epoxyeicosatetraenoic acids. Prior to labour, endogenous arachidonic acid metabolism in the amnion is principally via the lipoxygenase enzyme pathways. With labour, there is an increase in arachidonic acid metabolism and a change in the ratio of COX to lipoxygenase metabolites in favour of synthesis of prostaglandin E_2[19]. The roles of the lipoxygenase metabolites of arachidonic acid within the uterus are unknown, although 5-HETE may play a role in pre-labour (Braxton–Hicks) contractions[20,21].

Prostaglandin synthesis requires liberation of the substrate arachidonic acid by the action of a phospholipase, usually phospholipase A_2. Two forms of cellular phospholipase A_2 have been identified in intrauterine tissues, $sPLA_2$, a small molecular weight enzyme with homology to secreted PLA_2 and a larger cytosolic enzyme, $cPLA_2$. We have shown that placental $sPLA_2$ greatly exceeds expression in foetal membranes and that there is no change in $sPLA_2$ expression within the uterus during pregnancy or with the onset of labour[22]. Skannal et al.[23] found that $cPLA_2$ activity in foetal membranes increases during pregnancy and is highest in anticipation of labour, becoming depleted after labour. This suggests that it is $cPLA_2$ and not $sPLA_2$ which mediates increases in substrate arachidonic acid availability in foetal membranes with the onset of labour.

Until recently it was phospholipase activity which was thought to be the limiting factor in prostaglandin production in foetal membranes. However, any stimulus to prostaglandin production must also increase the activity of COX since it has a short half life and undergoes destruction after a limited number of reactions[24]. Our evidence that amnion produces predominately lipoxygenase metabolites of arachidonic acid before labour, and the change in the ratio of COX: lipoxygenase metabolism with labour, suggest that the activities of the two enzymes, COX and phospholipase, must be independently controlled[19,25]. There are two COX genes, the constitutively expressed COX-1 and the inducible COX-2[26,27].

In sheep the principal source of prostaglandins in late gestation is the placental cotyledon[28,29] and upregulation of COX-2 expression takes place gradually as pregnancy advances and precedes the labour-associated peak of maternal oestrogen concentrations. COX-1 expression within the sheep uterus does not change with gestational age[30,31].

In the human the principal sources of uterine prostaglandins are the foetal membranes and myometrium. We have used in situ hybridization to show expression of COX-1 and COX-2 in the foetal membranes[32]. Expression of COX-2 is mainly within the amnion epithelial layer and also in the cells of the amnionic mesoderm, reticular layer of the chorion and the decidua (Figure 1). COX-2 is not expressed in the trophoblast layer of the chorion. COX-1 expression is more diffuse throughout the foetal membranes, in the amnionic epithelium, amnionic mesoderm and also in the chorionic mesoderm and decidua. Using RT-PCR we have found that in amnion at term the COX-2 mRNA has over two orders of magnitude greater abundance than the COX-1 mRNA, whilst in myometrium the two isoforms are expressed at similar levels of mRNA abundance[32,33]. Hirst et al.[34] made similar findings using ribonuclease protection assays. We have found that COX-1 expression does not change with gestational age within the uterus. COX-2 expression increases in each tissue with gestational age and increases

Figure 1 Localization of human COX-2 in amnion–chorion rolls using in situ hybridization. Left panel, light field; right panel, dark field. Original magnification ×100. COX-2 expression can be seen in the amnion epithelium and sub-epithelial layer and in the decidua but not in the chorion (Slater et al. 1995, reference 32).

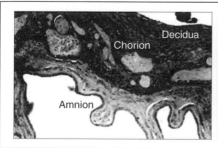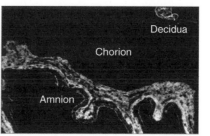

again with the onset of labour[35]. Enzyme kinetic studies of the human amnion[36] suggest that the increase in COX activity with the onset of labour is due entirely to an increase in the synthesis of the COX enzyme.

It is likely that the fundamental mechanisms controlling the switch from the pro-pregnancy to the pro-labour state is foetal in origin and has some relationship to foeto-placental size or maturity. Both McLean et al.[37] and Challis et al.[38] have suggested that the timing of labour is mediated through placental release of corticotrophin-releasing hormone (CRH) whose concentration in maternal plasma begins to rise about 90 days prior to the onset of labour. At 20 days prior to delivery, i.e. at about 37 weeks in the average pregnancy, CRH concentrations begin to exceed concentrations of the CRH-binding protein (Figure 2). The increase in COX-2 expression in amnion and chorion–decidua that we have shown, mirrors that of maternal CRH. CRH stimulates prostaglandin synthesis in foetal membranes[39] and in cultured decidua[40], possibly through upregulation of COX-2 expression. The increase in COX-2 expression in amnion after 38 weeks is more dramatic than in myometrium or chorion–decidua. Myometrium and chorion–decidua have a maternal blood supply and are therefore in contact with circulating factors including CRH. Amnion is avascular but is in contact

Figure 2 Changes in carticotrophin-releasing hormone (CRH) and corticotrophin-releasing hormone binding protein (CRH-BP) concentrations in maternal serum (adapted from McLean et al. 1995, reference 37) compared to COX-2 expression in amnion by RT-PCR.

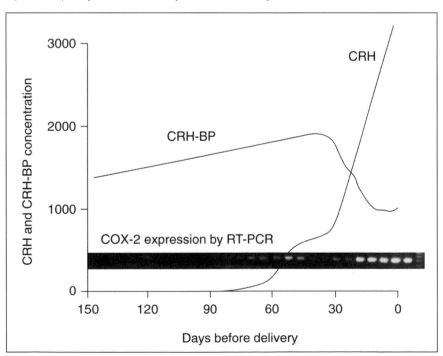

with the amniotic fluid. It has been suggested that a foetal stimulus may act to increase prostaglandin synthesis in amnion via the amniotic fluid. Candidates include platelet activating factor (PAF) whose concentration is related to foetal lung maturity[41] and interleukin (IL)-1[42,43] which may be transferred from the chorion–decidua, across the foetal membranes[44]. Myometrial and chorion–decidual COX-2 may therefore be upregulated by circulating factors such as CRH whilst the amnion could also be influenced by factors present in amniotic fluid such as PAF and IL-1β.

Although maternal oestrogen concentrations do not rise acutely before human labour, as they do in the sheep, there is a gradual rise in oestriol and oestradiol concentrations during the third trimester, reaching a plateaux at about 38 weeks[45]. The human placenta does not express the 17α-hydroxylase enzyme whose upregulation in sheep placenta causes the labour-associated rise in maternal oestrogens. Mecenas et al.[46] have suggested, however, that in primates, increased oestrogen synthesis prior to labour is mediated by increased availability of foetally-derived androgen substrates. Modest increases in primate maternal plasma oestrogens may reflect more dramatic changes in concentration locally within the uterus. Oestradiol upregulates oxytocin receptors and oxytocin synthesis within the uterus[47]. It does not, however, directly stimulate prostaglandin synthesis in pre-labour amnion[48] or in chorion[49]. Oestradiol increases prostaglandin synthesis in amnion collected following labour[48]; however, this may be secondary to stimulation of oxytocin synthesis and the increased oxytocin receptor density in amnion following labour. Challis et al.[38] suggest that placental CRH may increase dihydroepiandrostenedione production within the foetus, via increased placental and foetal ACTH. It is possible that CRH directly upregulates COX but upregulates other pro-labour genes such as the oxytocin receptor indirectly via foetal androgens and oestrogen. The mechanism of the onset of labour would therefore be similar in the human and the sheep, but with the secondary oestrogen-mediated stimulation of 'pro-labour' factors occurring less acutely.

PRE-TERM DELIVERY AND INCREASED COX-2 EXPRESSION

Pre-term delivery accounts for 10–15% of all live births and is the cause of 75% of neonatal morbidity and mortality. The cost of neonatal intensive care is over £1000 per day. At gestational ages below 28 weeks each day of prolongation of pregnancy increases survival rates by 5% and reduces the duration of neonatal intensive care by an average of two days.

Pre-term labour is multifactorial. The biochemistry underlying the various causes is gradually becoming understood. Most theories for the biochemical aetiology of pre-term labour have, as an important endpoint, increased prostaglandin synthesis mediated via increased COX-2 expression. Early pre-term labour is generally due to genital tract infection. Bacteria do not synthesize prostaglandins themselves[50] but increase prostaglandin synthesis both by release of phospholipase

A[20,25] and via lipopolysaccharide (LPS)-induced upregulation of COX-2 expression. We have shown that LPS increases prostaglandin synthesis in foetal membranes and increases COX-2 expression. Cervical incompetence may also lead to pre-term labour, through mechanical failure, by exposing the foetal membranes to the vagina and to stretch and by allowing bacteria access to the amniotic cavity. Pre-term labour may also occur through failure to metabolize the low concentrations of prostaglandins produced in the foetal membranes during pregnancy. Van Meir et al.[51] have shown deficient chorionic prostaglandin dehydrogenase activity associated with preterm labour both with and without infection.

Pre-term labour due to multiple pregnancy is probably due to increased placental mass, so that the critical CRH concentration which upregulates COX-2 synthesis is reached at an earlier gestational age. COX-2 and other contraction-associated proteins are stretch dependent, which may also contribute to early delivery in multiple pregnancy and hydramnios. Where there is foetal growth retardation or placental dysfunction, increased foetal cortisol will upregulate placental CRH synthesis[38] leading to a premature increase in COX-2 expression and the onset of pre-term labour.

NON-STEROIDAL ANTI-INFLAMMATORY DRUGS AND PRE-TERM LABOUR

The most commonly used tocolytics, beta-sympathomimetics, exhibit tachyphylaxis and can only delay delivery by 24 to 48 hours. Their use, in isolation, has no effect on perinatal morbidity although they have value in delaying delivery to allow in utero transfer to a tertiary unit or for administration of steroids to improve foetal pulmonary maturity. Beta-sympathomimetics are associated with potentially life threatening maternal side effects including disordered glucose tolerance, fluid retention, pulmonary oedema and heart failure. Calcium channel blockers are no more effective than beta-sympathomimetics although they may have fewer side effects. Magnesium sulphate is widely used in the USA but is no better than placebo. Oxytocin inhibitors are in clinical trial stages and appear to be effective in prevention of late, but not early pre-term labour. The only drug which has been shown, in randomized trials, to delay delivery for longer than 48 hours is indomethacin[52]. Indomethacin and other non-steroidal anti-inflammatory drugs (NSAIDs) are associated with unwanted foetal side effects, principally oligohydramnios and premature closure of the ductus arteriosus, which limit their use[53,54]. These are thought to be mediated by inhibition of COX-1, expressed constitutively in the affected foetal tissues. We have shown that COX-1 expression exceeds that of COX-2 in key foetal tissues including heart, kidney and brain, although these studies have been limited to before 24 weeks because of difficulties in obtaining tissues for study from later in pregnancy.

The use of a COX-2-selective NSAID should have the efficacy of indomethacin without the foetal side effects. Several new COX-2 selective

NSAIDs have been developed, but there is no experience of their use in pregnancy. Only two drugs with COX-2 selectivity are currently available for clinical use. These are meloxicam and nimesulide, each of which shows 10–100-fold selectivity for COX-2, depending upon the assay conditions.

We have found that nimesulide is as effective in inhibiting prostaglandin synthesis as non-COX-2-specific NSAIDs (Figure 3) and it effectively abolishes myometrial contractility (Figure 4). When administered intravenously to sheep in established labour nimesulide effectively stops uterine contractions and also appears to reverse the process of cervical ripening (Nathanielsz PW, personal communication). We have administered nimesulide to pregnant women at high risk of pre-term delivery[55] (Figure 5). The only foetal side effect which we have

Figure 3 Effect upon prostaglandin synthesis by IL-1β-stimulated human foetal membranes after incubation with various concentrations of COX-2 specific and non-specific NSAIDs. Tissue culture was for 24 hours.

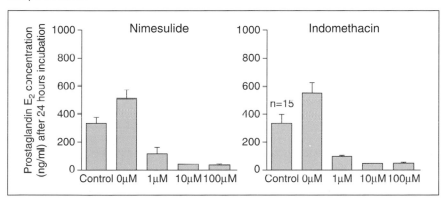

Figure 4 Contractility in two myometrial strips from the same patient, established in organ baths simultaneously. The top strip was treated with increasing concentrations of nimesulide, the bottom strip with vehicle only.

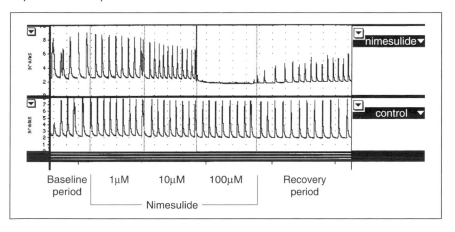

Figure 5 Amniotic fluid index measured as the sum of the deepest vertical pools in each of the four quadrants of the uterus during treatment with nimesulide, 200 mg daily. Dotted lines indicate the normal range of 5 to 25.

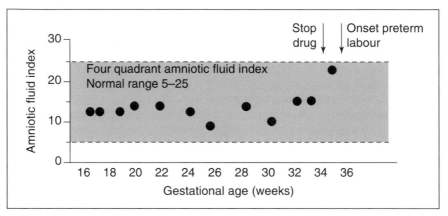

identified is oligohydramnios which occurs in approximately 50% of cases and after several weeks of administration. In our experience indomethacin treatment causes foetal side effects within 48–72 hours. It is possible that the foetal side effects that we see in women treated with nimesulide are due to drug accumulation in the foetus and the relatively high anti-COX-1 activity. Meloxicam may be an alternative with a half life suitable for once daily dosing and hence a smoother plasma concentration curve. At present COX-2-selective drugs with little or no anti-COX-1 activity are not available for use in pregnancy, but as they become available they will probably represent a major advance in the prevention of pre-term delivery.

REFERENCES

1. von Euler US. Uber die spezifische blutdrucksekende Substanz des menschlichen Prostata und Samenblasensekretes. *Klin Wochenschr.* 1934;14:1182–3.
2. Hawkins DF, Labrum AH. Semen prostaglandin levels in fifty patients attending a fertility clinic. *J Reprod Fertil.* 1961;2:1–10.
3. Sirois J. Induction of prostaglandin endoperoxide synthase-2 by human chorionic gonadotrophin in bovine preovulatory follicles in vivo. *Endocrinology.* 1994;135:841–8.
4. Kennedy TG. Evidence of a role for prostaglandins in the initiation of blastocyst implantation in the rat. *Biol Reprod.* 1977;16:286–91.
5. Chakraborty I, Das SK, Wang J, Dey SK. Developmental expression of the cyclo-oxygenase-1 and cyclo-oxygenase-2 genes in the peri-implantation mouse uterus and their differential regulation by the blastocyst and ovarian steroids. *J Mol Endocrinol.* 1996;16:107–22.
6. Coceani F, Bishai I, Bodach E, White EP, Olley PM. On the evidence implicating PGE$_2$ rather than prostacyclin in the patency of the fetal ductus arteriosus. In: Vane JR, Bergström S, editors. *Prostacyclin.* New York, Raven Press; 1979:247–52.
7. Langenbach R, Morham SG, Tiano SF, Loftin CD, Ghanaem BI, Chulada PC et al.

Prostaglandin synthase 1 gene disruption in mice reduces arachidonic acid-induced inflammation and indomethacin-induced gastric ulceration. *Cell.* 1995;83:483–92.

8. Morham SG, Langenbach R, Loftin CD, Tiano HF, Voloumanos N, Jenette C et al. Prostaglandin synthase 2 gene disruption causes severe renal pathology in the mouse. *Cell.* 1995;83:473–82.

9. Nguyen MT, Camenisch T, Snouwaert JN, Hicks E, Coffman TM, Anderson PAW et al. The prostaglandin receptor EP_4 triggers remodelling of the cardiovascular system at birth. *Nature.* 1997;390:78–81.

10. Sugimoto Y, Yamasaki A, Segi E, Tsuboi K, Aze Y, Nishimura T et al. Failure of parturition in mice lacking the prostaglandin F receptor. *Science.* 1997;277:681–3.

11. Lim H, Paria BC, Das SK, Dinchuk KE, Langenbach R, Trzackos JM et al. Multiple female reproductive failures in cyclooxygenase-2 deficient mice. *Cell.* 1997;91:197–208.

12. Challis JRG, Brookes AN. Maturation and activation of hypothalamic-pituitary function in fetal sheep. *Endocr Rev.* 1989;10:182–204.

13. Tangelakis K, Coghlan JP, Connell J. Tissue distribution and levels of gene expression of three steroid hydroxylases in ovine fetal adrenal gland. *Acta Endocrinol.* 1989;120:225–32.

14. Turnbull AC. *The Fetus and Birth.* London: Elsevier; 1977.

15. Skinner KA, Challis JRG. Changes in synthesis and metabolism of prostaglandins by human fetal membranes and decidua at labor. *Am J Obstet Gynecol.* 1985;151:519–23.

16. Crankshaw DJ, Dyal R. Effects of some naturally occurring prostanoids and some cyclo-oxygenase inhibitors on the contractility of the human lower uterine segment in vitro. *Can J Physiol Pharmacol.* 1994;72:870–4.

17. Liggins GC. Initiation of labour. *Biol Neonat.* 1989;55:366–75.

18. Garfield RE, Tabb T, Thilander G. Intercellular coupling and modulation of uterine contractility. In: Garfield RE, editor: *Uterine Contractility.* 1990 Serono Symposia New York, USA.

19. Bennett PR, Slater D, Elder MG, Moore GE. Changes in arachidonic acid metabolism in amnion cells associated with increased cyclo-oxygenase gene expression at parturition. *Br J Obstet Gynaecol.* 1993;100:1037–42.

20. Bennett PR, Elder MG, Myatt L. The effects of lipoxygenase metabolites of arachidonic acid upon contractility of human pregnant myometrium in vitro. *Prostaglandins.* 1988;33:837–44.

21. Walsh SW. 5-Hydroxyeicosatetraenoic acid, leukotriene C_4 and prostaglandin $F_{2\alpha}$ in amniotic fluid before and during term and preterm labor. *Am J Obstet Gynecol.* 1989;161:1352–60.

22. Slater DM, Dennes WJB, Sawdy R, Davies V, Bennett PR. Cyclo-oxygenase 2-selective NSAI drugs for inhibition of preterm labour. *Prostaglandins Leukot Essent Fatty Acids.* 1997;57:AM11.

23. Skannal DG, Brockman DE, Eis ALW, Xue S, Siddiqi TA, Myatt L. Changes in activity of cytosolic phospholipase A_2 in human amnion at term. *Am J Obstet Gynecol.* 1977;177:179–84.

24. Marshall PJ, Kulmacz RJ, Lands WEM. Constraints on prostaglandin synthesis in tissues. *J Biol Chem.* 1987;262:3510–7.

25. Bennett PR, Rose M, Myatt L, Elder MG. Preterm labor; stimulation of arachidonic acid metabolism in human amnion cells by bacterial products. *Am J Obstet Gynecol.* 1987;156:649–55.

26. Hla T, Farrell M, Kumar A, Bailey JM. Isolation of the cDNA for human prostaglandin H synthase. *Prostaglandins.* 1986;32:829–45.

27. O'Banion MK, Sadowski HB, Winn W, Young DA. A serum and glucocorticoid regulated 4kb mRNA encodes a cyclo-oxygenase-related protein. *J Biol Chem.* 1991;266:23261–7.

28. Mitchell MD, Flint A. Concentrations of prostaglandins in intrauterine tissues from late pregnant sheep before and after labour. *Prostaglandins.* 1977;14:563–9.
29. Rice GE, Wong MH, Thorburn GD. Gestational changes in prostaglandin synthase activity of cotyledonary microsomes. *J Endocrinol.* 1988;118:265–70.
30. Wimsatt J, Nathanielsz PW, Sirois J. Induction and prostaglandin endoperoxide synthase isoform-2 in ovine cotyledonary tissues during late gestation. *Endocrinology.* 1993;133:1068–73.
31. Rice GE, Freed KA, Aitken MA, Jacobs RA. Gestational and labour associated changes in relative abundance of prostaglandin G/H synthase-1 and -2 mRNA in ovine placenta. *J Mol Endocrinol.* 1995;14:237–44.
32. Slater DM, Berger L, Newton R, Moore GE, Bennett PR. Changes in the expression of types 1 and 2 cyclo-oxygenase in human fetal membranes at term. *Am J Obstet Gynecol.* 1995;172:77–82.
33. Slater DM, Berger L, Newton R, Moore GE, Bennett PR. The relative abundance of type 1 to type 2 cyclo-oxygenase mRNA in human amnion at term. *Biochem Biophys Res Commun.* 1994;198:304–8.
34. Hirst JJ, Teixeira FJ, Zakar T, Olson DM. Prostaglandin H synthase-2 expression increases in human gestational tissues with spontaneous labour onset. *Reprod Fertil Dev.* 1995;7:633–7.
35. Slater DM, Dennes WJB, Jones GD, Poston L, Bennett PR. Expression of COX-1 and COX-2 in myometrium. Changes in relation to gestation age and labour onset. *J Soc Gynecol Investig.* 1997;(suppl 4):A146.
36. Smieja Z, Zakar T, Waton JC, Olson DM. Prostaglandin endoperoxide synthase kinetics in human amnion before and after labour at term and following preterm labour. *Placenta.* 1993;14:163–75.
37. McLean M, Bisits A, Davies J, Woods R, Lowry P, Smith R. A placental clock controlling the length of human pregnancy. *Nature Medicine.* 1995;1:460–3.
38. Challis JRG, Matthews SG, Van Meir C, Ramirez MM. Current topic: The placental corticotrophin-releasing hormone-adrenocorticotrophin axis. *Placenta.* 1995;16:481–502.
39. Jones SA, Challis JR. Effects of corticotrophin-releasing hormone and adrenocorticotrophin on prostaglandin output by human placenta and fetal membranes. *Gynecol Obstet Invest.* 1990;29:165–8.
40. Petraglia F, Benedetto C, Florio P, D'Ambrigio G, Gennazzani AD, Marozio L et al. Effect of corticotrophin releasing factor binding protein on prostaglandin release from cultured maternal decidua and on contractile activity of human myometrium in vitro. *J Clin Endocrinol Metab.* 1995;80:3073–6.
41. Hoffman DR, Romero R, Johnston JM. Detection of platelet activating factor in amniotic fluid of complicated pregnancies. *Am J Obstet Gynecol.* 1990;162:525–8.
42. Romero R, Brody DT, Oyarzun E, Mazor M, Wu YK, Hobbins JC et al. Infection and labour III: IL-1: a signal for the onset of parturition. *Am J Obstet Gynecol.* 1989;160:1117–23.
43. Romero R, Drum S, Dinarello CA, Oyarzun E, Hobbins JC, Mitchell MD. IL-1β stimulates prostaglandin biosynthesis by human amnion. *Prostaglandins.* 1989; 37:13–22.
44. Kent AS, Sullivan MH, Elder MG. Transfer of cytokines through human fetal membranes. *J Reprod Fertil.* 1994;100:81–4.
45. Buster JE, Chang RJ, Preston DL, Elashoff RM, Cousins LM, Abraham GE et al. Interrelationships of circulating maternal steroid concentrations in third trimester pregnancies. *J Clin Endocrinol Metab.* 1978;48:133–44.
46. Mecenas CA, Giussani DA, Owiny JR, Jenkins SL, Wu WX, Honnebier BO et al. Production of premature delivery in pregnant rhesus monkeys by androstenedione infusion. *Nature Medicine.* 1996;2:443–8.

47. Fuchs AR, Periyasamy S, Alexandrova M, Soloff MS. Correlation between oxytocin receptor concentration and responsiveness to oxytocin in pregnant rat myometrium: Effects of ovarian steroids. *Endocrinology.* 1983;113:742–9.

48. Olson DM, Skinner K, Challis JR. Estradiol 17 beta and 2 hydroxyestradiol 17 beta induced differential production of prostaglandins by cells dispersed from human intrauterine tissues at parturition. *Prostaglandins.* 1983;25:639–51.

49. Gibb W, Riopel L, Collu R, Ducharme JR, Mitchell MD, Lavoie JC. Cyclo-oxygenase products formed by primary cultures of cells from human chorion laeve; influence of steroids. *Can J Physiol Pharmacol.* 1988;66:788–93.

50. Bennett PR, Elder MG. The mechanisms of preterm labor: common genital tract pathogens do not metabolize arachidonic acid to prostaglandins or to other eicosanoids. *Am J Obstet Gynecol.* 1992;166:1541–5.

51. van Meir CA, Sangha RK, Walton JC, Mathews SG, Keirse MJNC, Challis JRG. Immunoreactive 15-hydroxyprostaglandin dehydrogenase (PGDH) is reduced in fetal membranes from patients at preterm delivery in the presence of infection. *Placenta.* 1996;17:291–7.

52. Keirse MJNC. Indomethacin tocolysis in preterm labour. In: *Pregnancy and Cochrane Database of Systematic Reviews*, No 04383, 1995. BMJ Publishing.

53. Hendricks SK, Smith JR, Moore DE, Brown ZA. Oligohydramnios associated with prostaglandin synthetase inhibitors in preterm labour. *Br J Obstet Gynaecol.* 1990;97:312–6.

54. Moise KJ. Effect of advancing gestational age on the frequency of fetal ductal constriction in association with maternal indomethacin use. *Am J Obstet Gynecol.* 1993;168:1350–3.

55. Sawdy R, Slater DM, Fisk NM, Edmonds DK, Bennett PR. Use of a cyclo-oxygenase type-2 selective NSAI to prevent preterm delivery *Lancet.* 1997;350:265–6.

18

Cyclooxygenase-2 in Alzheimer's disease

M. K. O'BANION

Alzheimer's disease (AD) is the most common form of dementia in our ageing population, affecting more than four million people in the USA. The disease generally presents with memory impairment, but over a 5 to 10 year period progresses to involve most cortical functions, consistent with pathological changes in many brain regions. These changes include neuronal and synaptic loss, the presence of intracellular cytoskeletal 'tangles' and extracellular accumulation of amyloid β (Aβ) peptide as 'plaques'. The presence of these last two markers in sufficient numbers establishes the neuropathological diagnosis of AD. In addition to these hallmark pathologies there is a marked inflammatory reaction characterized by glial activation and endogenous expression of pro-inflammatory cytokines, MHC class II markers, complement components and acute phase reactant proteins[1,2]. These changes are consistently observed in AD brain tissue and appear to result, at least in part, from microglial and astrocytic reaction to Aβ deposition[3–5].

Numerous epidemiological studies and at least one small clinical trial indicate that non-steroidal anti-inflammatory drugs (NSAIDs) may slow the progression and delay the onset of AD (reviewed in reference 6). In 1989, Jenkinson et al.[7] reported that AD was less prevalent in patients with rheumatoid arthritis than in the general population. In a more extensive study of this association, McGeer et al.[8] were the first to suggest that the negative association of rheumatoid arthritis and AD might be due to the significant use of anti-inflammatory agents in this population. Similar associations have been found in case-controlled studies. For example, in siblings from families at high risk for AD, Breitner et al. demonstrated a significant delay (as much as 10 years) in the onset of AD symptoms with sustained prior NSAID use[9]. Rich et al.[10] found that AD patients taking NSAIDs performed better on cognitive tests and, relative to those not taking NSAIDs, showed less decline over a one year period in verbal fluency, spatial recognition and orientation. Finally, Stewart et al.[11] provided the first *prospective* evaluation of NSAID therapy for delaying AD. These investigators found a relative risk of 0.40 for persons with two or more years of NSAID use prior to disease onset. Importantly, they found no significant effect with aspirin or paracetamol. In addition to these epidemiological studies, Rogers and colleagues demonstrated that 14 AD patients treated for six months with indomethacin showed a slight improvement in tests of cognitive function, whereas 14 patients receiving placebo showed a decline[12].

Based on the findings of an inflammatory reaction in AD tissue and the apparent benefits of NSAIDs in slowing the progression or delaying the onset of AD, we and others have postulated that cyclooxygenase (COX) plays a role in the disease. As set out below, our results to date suggest two potential mechanisms for the pathological involvement of COX-2 in AD. In the first, glial expression of COX-2 plays an important role in the elaboration of inflammatory changes, similar to the role of COX-2 in peripheral inflammation. An alternative possibility is that neuronal COX-2 expression contributes to the death of neurones.

ASTROCYTES EXPRESS COX-2 IN RESPONSE TO PRO-INFLAMMATORY CYTOKINES

We reported previously that prostaglandin $(PG)E_2$ levels increased over time in primary cultures of mouse astrocytes treated with the pro-inflammatory cytokine interleukin-1β (IL-1β). Concurrent treatment with dexamethasone abrogated this response, suggesting that prostanoid production was due to increased levels of COX-2[13]. Northern blot analysis revealed a time- and dose-dependent elevation of COX-2 mRNA in cells treated with IL-1β. Also we found increased levels of COX-2 mRNA after two hours in cultures treated with tumour necrosis factor-α, phorbol ester and basic fibroblast growth factor, indicating that many factors have the ability to regulate COX-2 in astrocytes[13]. We confirmed that elevations in COX-2 message correlated with increased COX activity that was inhibited by the selective COX-2 inhibitor NS-398[14]. Induction of COX-2 protein in cultured astrocytes is shown in Figure 1. Also, we have observed COX-2 induction following IL-1β treatment of rat astrocytes[15] and have preliminary data that human astrocytes make COX-2 in response to IL-1β. Similar findings have been reported by others in ovine astrocytes[16].

Microglia represent the resident macrophages of the central nervous system, and several investigators have demonstrated induction of COX-2 in cultured microglia by lipopolysaccharide[17,18]. Microglia and astrocytes undergo specific morphological and biochemical changes following brain trauma, ischaemia or neurodegeneration. This activation process is associated with the expression of pro-inflammatory cytokines and acute phase reactant proteins. Based on in vitro studies it seems likely that COX-2 will play a role in the elaboration of these

Figure 1 *COX-2 induction in cultured mouse astrocytes. Astrocytes were treated with (a) 0.1% dimethylsulphoxide (control) or (b) 100 nM phorbol ester for six hours, fixed briefly with 4% paraformaldehyde, and immunostained using a monoclonal antibody raised to human COX-2 (Transduction Laboratories, Lexington, KY, USA). Standard avidin–biotin enhancement was carried out and diaminobenzidine was used as the chromogen. 20× objective.*

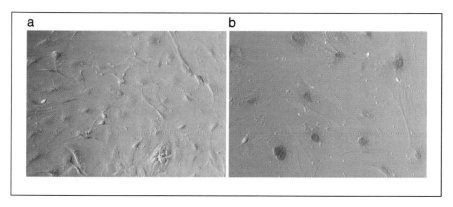

changes. For example, Fiebich and colleagues have demonstrated that IL-6 is induced by PGE_2 in a human astrocytoma cell line[19]. Despite strong evidence in tissue culture models, to date there are few data demonstrating glial COX-2 expression in vivo. Nevertheless, the idea that AD pathogenesis involves inflammatory changes mediated by glial COX-2 remains an attractive hypothesis.

NEURONES EXPRESS COX-2 IN RESPONSE TO SYNAPTIC ACTIVATION

In 1993, Yamagata and colleagues[20] demonstrated that COX-2 was induced as an immediate early gene in cortical and hippocampal neurones following electrically induced seizures. Also they showed that neuronal COX-2 expression was regulated by physiologically relevant stimuli and glucocorticoids. Additional studies revealed a developmental profile for COX-2 expression corresponding to a critical period of cortical synapse formation[21]. Kaufmann et al. demonstrated that COX-2 was expressed in glutamatergic neurones and localized to both the cell body and dendrites[21]. We have made similar observations in rats subjected to seizures induced by peripheral injection of the excitotoxin, kainic acid. As shown in Figure 2, COX-2 immunoreactivity in the rat hippocampus is dramatically increased after 24 hours and remains elevated for 72 hours following seizure induction. COX-2 is readily detected in dendrites as shown by strong staining of the molecular (dendritic) layer of the dentate gyrus in seizured animals (Figure 2b and c) and in cortical neurones in control rats (Figure 2d).

Other investigators have reported induction of COX-2 mRNA in neurones following kainic acid treatment, intracerebral injection of an excitotoxin or ischaemia[22-26]. Direct support for COX-2 contributing to neuronal demise comes

Figure 2 *COX-2 immunoreactivity is dramatically enhanced in rat neurones following kainate-induced seizures and localizes to the cell body and dendrites. Forty-micron sections prepared from 4% paraformaldehyde-fixed rat brain were immunostained with a monoclonal antibody raised to human COX-2 (Transduction Laboratories, Lexington, KY, USA). Standard avidin–biotin enhancement was carried out and diaminobenzidine was used as the chromogen. The dentate gyrus cells of the hippocampus are shown in (a) control and (b) 24 hours and (c) 72 hours following induction of seizures. In (b) and (c) note intense staining for COX-2 in the dendritic arborization (molecular layer; ml) of the dentate gyrus, 2.5× objective. (d) Shows neurones in the cortex of a control rat, 20× objective.*

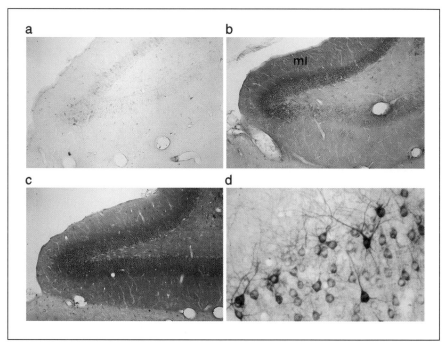

from a study by Nogawa et al. These investigators showed COX-2 induction in neurones following focal ischaemia and found a significant neuroprotective effect when rats were treated with NS-398[27]. The expression of COX-2 in neurones and the demonstration of neuroprotection with a selective COX-2 inhibitor cannot be ignored in consideration of prominent neuronal cell loss in AD[28].

COX-2 EXPRESSION IN AD

To begin to characterize the potential role of COX-2 in AD we have carried out studies of COX expression in postmortem human tissue from control and AD patients. In a small number of cases we reported a decrease in brain COX-2 mRNA levels in AD and observed COX-2 mRNA in neurones by in situ hybridization[15]. Unfortunately, we have not been able to replicate these findings, despite numerous attempts. The reasons for this are not clear, but a recent report by Lukiw and Bazan[29] indicates that COX-2 mRNA is not stable in postmortem tissue. Thus, COX-2 mRNA does not appear to represent an ideal marker for studies in human brain. A report of increased COX-2 protein in AD has been presented in abstract form[30]. Another group reported COX-2 immunostaining in tangle-bearing neurones of AD and Down's syndrome patients[31]. We have not been able to reproduce these later findings, using several antibodies that detect human COX-2 on immunoblots (data not shown). Additional studies using optimized immunostaining protocols are in progress.

COX-1 IS UPREGULATED IN A MODEL OF NEURONAL DIFFERENTIATION

It is important to keep in mind that COX-1 is also expressed in the nervous system[32]. The PC12 cell line was derived from a rat phaeochromocytoma and is widely used as a model of neuronal differentiation. When treated with nerve growth factor (NGF), these cells stop dividing, extend neurites and express genes important for neurotransmitter biosynthesis[33]. NGF-induced differentiation of PC12 cells also leads to increased production of prostanoids[34]. As shown in Figure 3, COX-1 protein levels are elevated in PC12 cells treated with NGF. In this example, cells were treated with various doses of NGF for four days. In other experiments, COX-1 mRNA levels were increased within six hours of NGF treatment and protein levels remained elevated for as long as 14 days[35]. These studies were the first to demonstrate regulation of COX expression by neuronotrophic factors.

Figure 3 NGF induces COX-1 in PC12 cells. In (a) PC12 cells were treated for four days with the indicated concentrations of NGF. Cell lysates were subject to Western blot analysis with an antibody that recognizes rat COX-1. In the lane on the far right, lysate was from cells treated with 50 ng/ml NGF that had been pre-incubated with 10-fold excess neutralizing anti-NGF antibody (αNGF). In (b) data are the mean laser densitometric values±S.E.M. (n = 4) of COX-1 protein levels relative to controls. **P<0.02 versus 50 ng/ml of NGF, two-tailed Student's t test. From reference 35 with permission.

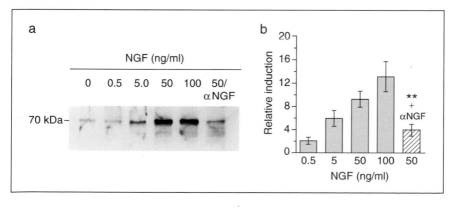

CONCLUSIONS

Epidemiological studies of NSAID use and AD provide support for the hypothesis that COX is involved in the pathogenesis of AD, but we do not yet understand the mechanism by which this occurs. Based on studies in tissue culture, animal models and human brain there are two models for COX-2 involvement; one related to glial expression and inflammation, the other to neuronal susceptibility. These models are not mutually exclusive. Also, it is possible that COX-1 is involved or that effects of NSAIDs in the periphery somehow influence the disease. Trials currently under way with selective COX-2 inhibitors may yield information about the isoform involved, at least in the progression of the disease. Although the epidemiological data suggest that people will benefit from long-term NSAID therapy, we have little clear information regarding the normal roles COX serves in the central nervous system. Evidence suggesting a developmental role for COX-2 and our demonstration that COX-1 is regulated by a neuronotrophic factor indicate that caution should be exercised before subjecting people to long-term therapies aimed at inhibiting brain COX activity.

Acknowledgements

I thank past and present members of my laboratory, including J. W. Chang, J. C. Dusel, M. D. Kaplan, S. Kyrkanides, J. Rollins and A. Yermakova, and my colleagues L. Callahan and J. Olschowka for their contributions to this work. This work was supported by grants from the NIH (NS33553, AG09016), the Rochester Alzheimer's Disease Center (AG08665) and the Lucille P. Markey Charitable Trust.

REFERENCES

1. McGeer P, McGeer E. The inflammation response system of the brain: implications for therapy of Alzheimer and other neurodegenerative diseases. *Brain Res Rev.* 1995;21:195–218.
2. Rogers J, O'Barr S. Inflammatory mediators in Alzheimer's disease. In: Wasco W, Tanzi RE, editors. *Molecular Mechanisms of Dementia.* Totowa, NJ: Humana Press, Inc.; 1997:177–98.
3. Griffin WST, Sheng JG, Mrak RE. Inflammatory pathways: implications in Alzheimer's disease. In: Wasco W, Tanzi RE, editors. *Molecular Mechanisms of Dementia.* Totowa, NJ: Humana Press, Inc.; 1997:169–76.
4. Cotman CW, Tenner AJ, Cummings BJ. β-Amyloid converts an acute phase injury response to chronic injury responses. *Neurobiol Aging.* 1996;17:723–31.
5. Rogers J, Webster S, Lue L-F, Brachova L, Civin WH, Emmerling M et al. Inflammation and Alzheimer's disease pathogenesis. *Neurobiol Aging.* 1996;17:681–6.
6. Breitner JCS. The role of anti-inflammatory drugs in the prevention and treatment of Alzheimer's disease. *Annu Rev Med.* 1996;47:401–11.
7. Jenkinson ML, Bliss MR, Brain AT, Scott DL. Rheumatoid arthritis and senile dementia of the Alzheimer's type. *Br J Rheumatol.* 1989;28:86–8.
8. McGeer PL, McGeer E, Rogers J, Sibley J. Anti-inflammatory drugs and Alzheimer disease.

Lancet. 1990;335:1037.

9. Breitner JCS, Welsh KA, Helms MJ, Gaskell PC, Gau BA, Roses AD et al. Delayed onset of Alzheimer's disease with nonsteroidal anti-inflammatory and histamine H_2 blocking drugs. *Neurobiol Aging*. 1995;16:523–30.

10. Rich JB, Rasmusson DX, Folstein MF, Carson KA, Kawas C, Brandt J. Nonsteroidal anti-inflammatory drugs in Alzheimer's disease. *Neurology*. 1995;45:51–5.

11. Stewart WF, Kawas C, Corrada M, Metter EJ. Risk of Alzheimer's disease and duration of NSAID use. *Neurology*. 1997;48:626–32.

12. Rogers J, Kirby LC, Hempelman SR, Berry DL, McGeer PL, Kaszniak AW et al. Clinical trial of indomethacin in Alzheimer's disease. *Neurology*. 1993;43:1609–11.

13. O'Banion MK, Dusel JC, Chang JW, Kaplan MD, Coleman PD. Interleukin-1β induces prostaglandin G/H synthase-2 (cyclooxygenase-2) in primary murine astrocyte cultures. *J Neurochem*. 1996;66:2532–40.

14. Futaki N, Takahashi S, Yokoyama M, Arai I, Higuchi S, Otomo S. NS-398, a new anti-inflammatory agent, selectively inhibits prostaglandin G/H synthase/cyclooxygenase (COX-2) activity in vitro. *Prostaglandins*. 1994;47:55–9.

15. Chang JW, Coleman PD, O'Banion MK. Prostaglandin G/H synthase-2 (cyclooxygenase-2) mRNA expression is decreased in Alzheimer's disease. *Neurobiol Aging*. 1996;17:801–8.

16. Thore CR, Nam MJ, Busija DW. Immunofluorescent localization of constitutive and inducible prostaglandin H synthase in ovine astroglia. *J Comp Neurol*. 1996;367:1–9.

17. Bauer MKA, Lieb K, Schulze-Osthoff K, Berger M, Gebicke-Haerter PJ, Bauer J et al. Expression and regulation of cyclooxygenase-2 in rat microglia. *Eur J Biochem*. 1997;243:726–31.

18. Minghetti L, Polazzi E, Nicolini A, Créminon C, Levi G. Interferon gamma and nitric oxide down-regulate lipopolysaccharide-induced prostanoid production in cultured rat microglial cells by inhibiting cyclooxygenase-2 expression. *J Neurochem*. 1996;66:1963–70.

19. Fiebich BL, Hüll M, Lieb K, Gyufko K, Berger M, Bauer J. Prostaglandin E_2 induces interleukin-6 synthesis in human astrocytoma cells. *J Neurochem*. 1997;68:704–9.

20. Yamagata K, Andreasson KI, Kaufmann WI, Barnes CA, Worley PF. Expression of a mitogen-inducible cyclooxygenase in brain neurons: regulation by synaptic activity and glucocorticoids. *Neuron*. 1993;11:371–86.

21. Kaufmann WE, Worley PF, Pegg J, Bremer M, Isakson P. Cox-2, a synaptically-induced enzyme, is expressed by excitatory neurons at postsynaptic sites in rat cerebral cortex. *Proc Natl Acad Sci USA*. 1996;93:2317–21.

22. Adams J, Collaço-Moraes Y, de Belleroche J. Cyclooxygenase-2 induction in cerebral cortex: an intracellular response to synaptic excitation. *J Neurochem*. 1996;66:6–13.

23. Chen J, Marsh T, Zhang JS, Graham SH. Expression of cyclooxygenase-2 in rat brain following kainate treatment. *Neuroreport*. 1995;6:245–8.

24. Miettinen S, Fusco FR, Yrjänheikki J, Hirvanen T, Raivanen R, Narhi M et al. Spreading depression and focal brain ischemia induce cyclooxygenase-2 in cortical neurons through N-methyl-D-aspartic acid receptors and phospholipase A_2. *Proc Natl Acad Sci USA*. 1997;94:6500–5.

25. Ohtsuki T, Kitagawa K, Yamagata K, Mandai K, Mabuchi T, Matsushita K et al. Induction of cyclooxygenase-2 mRNA in gerbil hippocampal neurons after transient forebrain ischemia. *Brain Res*. 1996;736:353–6.

26. Toco G, Freiremoar J, Schreiber SS, Sakhi SH, Aisen PS, Pasinetti GM. Maturational regulation and regional induction of cyclooxygenase-2 in rat brain – implications for Alzheimer's disease. *Exp Neurol*. 1997;144:339–49.

27. Nogawa S, Zhang F, Ross ME, Iadecola C. Cyclooxygenase-2 gene expression in neurons contributes to ischemic brain damage. *J Neurosci*. 1997;17:2746–55.

28. O'Banion MK, Coleman PD, Callahan LM. Regional neuronal loss in aging and Alzheimer's disease: a brief review. *Semin Neurosci.* 1994;6:307–14.

29. Lukiw WJ, Bazan NG. Cyclooxygenase 2 RNA message abundance, stability, and hypervariability in sporadic Alzheimer neocortex. *J Neurosci Res.* 1997;50:937–45.

30. Wei Y, Aisen PS, Freire-Moar J, Whiteley P, Swinney DC, Mak AY et al. Cyclooxygenase-2 in Alzheimer's disease brain. *Soc Neurosci Abstr.* 1997;23:1632.

31. Oka A, Takashima S. Induction of cyclooxygenase 2 in brains of patients with Down's syndrome and dementia of the Alzheimer's type: specific localization in affected neurones and axons. *Neuroreport.* 1997;8:1161–4.

32. Breder CD, Smith WL, Raz A, Masferrer JL, Seibert K, Needleman P et al. Distribution and characterization of cyclooxygenase immunoreactivity in the ovine brain. *J Comp Neurol.* 1992;322:409–38.

33. Greene LA, Aletta JM, Rukenstein A, Green SH. PC12 pheochromocytoma cells: culture, nerve growth factor treatment, and experimental exploitation. *Methods Enzymol.* 1987;147:207–16.

34. DeGeorge JJ, Walenga R, Carbonetto S. Nerve growth factor rapidly stimulates arachidonate metabolism in PC12 cells: potential involvement in nerve fiber growth. *J Neurosci Res.* 1988;21:323–32.

35. Kaplan MD, Olschowka JA, O'Banion MK. Cyclooxygenase-1 behaves as a delayed response gene in PC12 cells differentiated by nerve growth factor. *J Biol Chem.* 1997;272:18534–7.

Index